*you can*

# TRUST YOURSELF

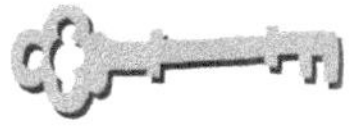

# you can TRUST YOURSELF

unlock the wise woman within
using modern tools + ancient wisdom

EMILY ROMERO, LPC, SEP

## ADVANCED PRAISE

**"*You Can Trust Yourself* is the book you needed to read yesterday!** Every page is filled with wisdom, practical advice and points of introspection that will leave you feeling like you just had tea with your wise and wonderful best friend (*if your bestie also invented a model for healing and was a total badass*). Every woman should read this."
••• Caitlan Siegenthaler, *IFS Therapist + Human Design Strategist*

**"If you've heard about *Internal Family Systems (IFS)* and are curious, *You Can Trust Yourself* is the perfect entry with a big impact.** This book is truly is the perfect amount to give you what you need to start integrating it into your own journey without feeling overwhelming. It's a gentle nudge to start getting curious about your own parts. I would highly recommend reading this book... and then reading it again."
••• Meghan Jaskinia, *The Monarch Evolution*

"The great Carl Jung said, "The privilege of a lifetime is to become who you truly are." *You Can Trust Yourself* is your roadmap to get there. An invitation to come home to yourself. **In a market saturated with self-help schemes, Emily's work in the world is infused with integrity and care.** This book is honest, vulnerable and meant for the hands of those ready to be the same."
••• Haley Smith, *Holistic Fertility Clinic*

"In a field dominated by male voices and masculine ideology, it is refreshing to have a resource created by a woman, for women. *You Can Trust Yourself* is relatable and **Emily is skillful as she weaves together her training and knowledge - saving you from getting a degree in psychology.** Reading this book felt like she was in my corner, supporting, challenging and validating me."

••• Journey Lee, *Complex Humxn Counseling*

"*You Can Trust Yourself* tackles a subject that baffles most of us daily... Self-Trust. And with her extensive knowledge, humor, and vulnerability, Emily has authored a brilliant depiction of her model for Self-Trust which **de-mystifies our inner worlds and invites us to believe in, well... ourSELVES!**"

••• Kathie Hoffmann, *Be Therapy, Etc*

"*You Can Trust Yourself* sucked me in like a beautiful hurricane! **The guidance of *The Self-Trust Compass* makes it easier to navigate the metaphorical seasons of life and find grace in the non-linear aspects of healing.** Her collection of ideas helps tap into the wisdom that transcends logic. I will definitely be keeping a few copies on hand to gift to friends!"

••• Lo Anzivino, *Spiritual Wellness Guide*

Cover Design: Emily Romero

Illustrations: Kasey Strobel

www.curiosityrising.com

For bulk order discounts: contact@curiosityrising.com

# DISCLAIMER

The names, stories, clients, and situations described in this book are composites of many individuals, drawn from both my experience and my colleagues' experiences. They are not meant to represent any specific person or event. The details have been changed and fictionalized to ensure the privacy and confidentiality of all involved. Any resemblance to actual persons, living or dead, is not intentional.

This book is intended for general information purposes only. Any application of the material set forth is to be used at the reader's discretion and is their sole responsibility.

This book is not endorsed by the creators of *Somatic Experiencing®* or *Internal Family Systems®*. All information shared is based off my interpretations from the trainings I've received. But if you want to put me in contact with their creators, I'd love to have them check this book out!

# DEDICATION

This is for the woman with a strong intuition...
but who still doubts herself.

This is for the woman who desires "more"...
but settles for "fine".

This is for the woman who deeply knows...
but second-guesses.

**This is for the woman who knows in her bones she's meant to return...to the path of trusting herself.**

# EXPECTATIONS

This book won't give you the answers.

But it will give you tools to discover *your* answers - for yourself.

# CONTENTS

# PROLOGUE

Let's begin our reader/author relationship with some mutual honesty. *I'll go first...*

I'm going to start this book explicitly with something I'm trying to do less of, but in this instance, an exception is warranted.

I'm going to offer you a disclaimer.

Ready? Here it is...

**This book might actually *not* be for you.**

Hear me out, so you can decide if you want to immediately return it to the same shelf you just picked it up from.

Or, if you want to block off the next few hours of your day to curl up with a warm drink and this 400+ page reminder of the wise and badass woman that you are.

I'm going to say a lot of things over the next few hundred pages. I'm going to offer you insight from many different therapeutic frameworks. I'm going to share a model I've created for you, as a guide. I'm going to include examples of ancient wisdom - rediscovered many times over. And, I'm going to offer you some modern tools so you can actually apply these learnings to your everyday life.

There will be times throughout this book that I'll treat you like one of my thousands of therapy clients over the years, by encouraging you to slow down, offering you different perspectives to consider, practices to try, and a few well timed moments of - answering your direct question... with a question. *Sorry, it's a habit I can't seem to kick.*

At other times, I'm going to pretend there is no way that you, dear reader, could possibly be a past client of mine. Because I'm also going to sprinkle in some personal stories that never would've gotten through my old "blank slate" vetting system. *Watch out, I might even share some of my journal entries with you.*

I'm going to say a lot of things over the next few hundred pages. But the single most important thing I'll say this entire time, is this one simple belief I have...

**I believe that YOU can trust yourself.**

*Even if it feels impossible to you right now.*

And, I also believe that knowing you have your own back in this way, might be the single most important thing you can ever learn to do. *Especially if it feels impossible to you right now.*

Now that you know what I believe, let's come back to the disclaimer.

This book might *not* be for you.

If connecting to yourself, your body, your intuition, your inner child, and your inner wisdom comes easy to you right now - *you probably don't need this book.*

There are a million free and simple ways to connect to your deepest knowing, your higher guidance, your soul's calling, or whatever language resonates with you. You don't need me (or anyone else) for that. *No matter what any "guru" or "self-help expert" tells you.*

If you hear someone say, *"Trust Your Gut"* and that's enough guidance for you - *take that advice and go live your best life.*

**This book is specifically for the woman who's struggling in the ways I was a decade or so ago:**

- It's for the woman who feels broken because the *"fake-it-till-you-make-it"* confidence strategy she's been told is the answer - doesn't seem to work long term.
- It's for the woman who thinks *"Just Trust Yourself!"* sounds nice - but doesn't know how to *actually* reach this elusive platitude.
- It's for the woman who knows her answers are inside *her* - but just needs a framework to guide and connect her back to the wisdom within.
- It's for the woman whose biggest antagonists are "Fear" & "Doubt".
- And... it's for the woman who doesn't *actually* like being told what to do.

**Now, it's your turn to be honest...**

> *Are you actually ready for what is required to get the life you say you want?*

You're probably not picking up a personal development book if everything in your life is *exactly* how you want it to be.

There is likely some aspect of your life that you want to be different.

Somewhere...change is calling.

The necessary change may look like the dramatic transformations you see in the movies. Moving across the country, quitting a job, ending a relationship, drastically changing your health habits, or going on a soul-searching trip around the world.

Or maybe, there's already a lot going *well* in your life. The change you desire might seem less extreme. Maybe you want to set different boundaries with your in-laws, maybe you want to approach your next pregnancy in a different way, maybe you want to travel more, or take up a new creative hobby. Maybe you want to ask for a raise. Maybe you've already done a ton of personal healing and it's just a few tweaks that are needed now.

No matter what change you desire in your life, be honest with yourself...

*Are you actually ready to do things in a different way?*

**The cool thing about this book is... it doesn't really matter what your answer is. It only matters that you're honest.**

If the answer is a *"Hell yes, I'm at the end of my rope, I have to do something different!"* - then great. You're in good company. Many women who have followed this approach have also recognized a calling within themselves to make changes. Sometimes, this was just the tipping point to do the thing they'd wanted to do for a long time. Some of them DID move across the country, quit their jobs, and leave the unhealthy relationships. If this is you, I'm going to encourage you to not just *read* this book...but to actually *apply* the lessons. Integrate the concepts into your daily life. Do the exercises. Try out the practices. See what resonates for you. **Play around with some "doing" energy.**

If the answer, instead, is some version of *"I don't know... maybe things aren't so bad... I think I'm probably fine."* - also great. This tells you your starting point. Maybe you're "Self-Trust Curious". That's perfect. You can still read this book. You can still tune into what resonates. You can pay attention to ideas and practices that scare you. You can **play around with the energy of "being"**. You don't have to do anything drastic. In fact, I encourage you to wait until you can't *not* do it.

This book is *not* meant to be a field guide in blowing up your life. You don't have to do anything you don't want to do.

Actually, as I write this now, I'm reminded of a thought I almost said many times to people as I was going through my divorce, when I noticed a *particular* look in their eyes. I wanted to reassure them...

*"Don't worry, divorce isn't contagious...*

*Unless you want it to be."*

[ 1 ]

# THE FALSE SUMMIT

January 23rd

It's done. We're done. I just finished hosting the second round of a multi-retreat program.

Season 2 of Adventure Club... is DONE.

I'm so grateful I took the leap to start this group and I honestly can't believe this is my life... This is actually the life I get to live.

No way 23-year-old-me would've believed it.

Here I am... the morning after such an incredible experience...

Physically exhausted. Spiritually electric.

Thinking about all the growth these women have gone through together...

The fears they faced in Portland... the inner work they navigated in Denver... and the life-long connections they solidified, here, in San Diego.

My body feels as relaxed as the palm trees swaying outside, both of us moving with the same slow rhythm.

THIS is the life I've always wanted...

A life of travel and adventure.

A life of "work" that consists of bringing together incredible women for hiking, surfing, tea ceremonies, transformative conversations, and plenty of laughing tears.

All of it - without the 50-minute time constraint of traditional therapy.

THIS is it.

THIS is the work I want to keep doing.

THIS feels... magical.

And while I can already feel the pull to start planning the next season, I know I need to slow down this time.

I allowed my excitement, and the eagerness of the women on the waitlist, to move me so quickly from the first season directly into the second. This time I want to remember to pause… and celebrate what we're creating together.

I want to remember to enjoy life as it's happening.

Plus, I only have two months left before I officially shut down my therapy practice. Two months left of working under my therapy license. Two months that will be full of hard goodbyes.

That's what I need to focus on.

That's what I need to be present for.

The next season of my business and my life will start in March.

And I can't freaking wait…

Because, if everything goes according to plan, the next season of life will be filled with much more of THIS.

# [ 2 ]
# META SELF-TRUST

Three months after I closed down my therapy practice, my profit & loss statement confirmed what I already knew to be true, but didn't want to acknowledge.

I'd been working my ass off to build my new group coaching business. And yet, in the first six months, I made less money than I used to make in one month of my therapy practice.

> *Remind me again why I left a career I loved?*
> *Remind me again why I shut down a business I worked so hard to build?*

I already knew the simple but annoying answer: I couldn't *not* do it.

I know now, all too well, the cost of ignoring my intuition when she speaks. And it's a price I'm no longer willing to pay. So now, when the inner whisper only I can hear comes through, I listen. I try not to wait for her to scream at me anymore.

But that doesn't mean she makes things easy on me, just because I listen. Following your intuition in life often leads to an expansive life, but not necessarily an easy life. Or even the one you would've expected. But I know myself well enough by now to know that when these two options are side by side, I'm not pushing the easy button now.

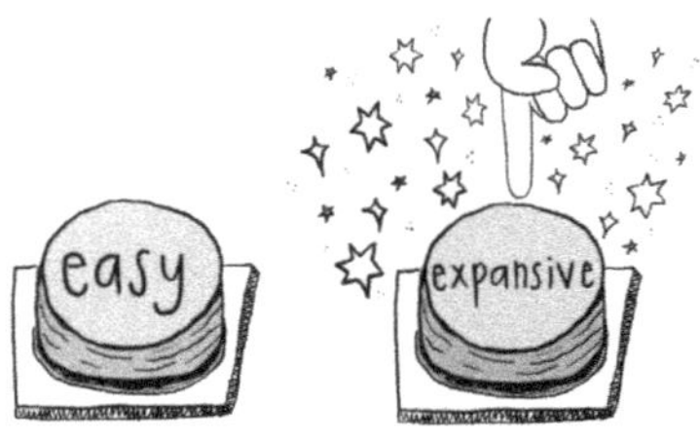


The decision to end my practice goes back further than my final session as a therapist. Six months earlier, I navigated what we could call a complicated inner family "discussion"...

A part of me was resistant to the change I felt coming. She was trying to hold onto my identity as a therapist (and the box it put me in). While other parts were ready to expand into the kind of work that truly lit me up and the mystery of what could unfold on the other side.

And the work that truly lit me up was still taking shape. My first experience of Self-Trust getting meta was in the creation of what would eventually be called, *Adventure Club.*

**It definitely wasn't group therapy. But it also wasn't a typical wellness retreat.**

I was exploring the edges and working outside my therapy license in a new and exciting way. And I brought together an intimate group of women to explore their own paths to trusting themselves more deeply.

The creation of this group on Self-Trust was, in and of itself, an act of Self-Trust. Doing the scary thing I couldn't *not* do. Trusting I didn't need every detail figured out ahead of time. I just needed to keep taking the next right step down the path I knew in my bones was right. One after another... after another.

We hiked, we laughed, we sat with tea, we cried, we explored the questions that tend to stay in the shadows. We ventured into spaces of trust - with ourselves and each other. All of it was lighting the fire in my soul. Looking back, it makes sense that it was only a matter of time before I needed to leap more fully into that world.

While still trying to juggle my individual therapy practice alongside this group coaching adventure, a message soon came through with clarity:

*"You need to close down your therapy practice."*

Because I know the consequences now, I listened. Maybe a little bit skeptically, but still I listened. And started taking action.

*The Self-Trust Model*™, which is what this entire book is about, formed from over 13 years as a somatic trauma therapist, as well as from my own personal life. But I'd never applied the model directly to my business before.

Five years in, I now have the experience of building a financially successful business, with multiple streams of income. I've been tested more personally in the past five years than my first three decades combined.

I've proven to myself, repeatedly, that I can trust myself.

And so, yeah, maaaaaaaybe I let some expectations creep in.

Expectations that this new business endeavor would be easier this time around. The onramp to success would be shorter.

But, you know what they say about expectations...

I found myself saying...

> *Shouldn't this be working by now?*
> *Shouldn't this be easier?*

Even though, I'm not as quick to listen to "Should" as I once was, she still makes some pretty convincing points. It was hard to *not* let a little doubt creep back in.

Especially because it's not *just* about the money.

Another aspect of why I decided to close my therapy practice was to have more time *away* from work. I wanted more spaciousness for family and creativity and fun. I wanted to *not* over-work for the first time in my life. I thought if I ended one of my full time jobs, and solely focused on the Self-Trust groups, I'd finally get that extra time.

But, as you might already be able to guess... that's not what happened.

Just as the profit & loss statement didn't lie, my calendar didn't either. I'd spent way more time working in the first months of my new business than I did when my therapy practice was at its peak. I was spending less time with family and creative projects than ever before.

And, on top of all of that, I was feeling really discouraged. Because I was spending most of my time doing things I wasn't good at. Back-end systems, technology, social media and marketing are exhausting to me. They are lightyears away from my superpowers. And while I know there are many important lessons that come from learning curves in business, it's also super defeating to spend most of your time doing things you're not good at.

*Something* had to change.

**Spoiler Alert: Something = Me**

Then, I watched myself as I taught inside one of my newest online groups. I listened to myself as I encouraged someone to come back to the basics. To make sure to build a solid foundation first, even when it's tempting to bypass to the new and shiny thing.

After I ended the video meeting, it was obvious. And I allowed my clarity and intuition to flow through the tip of my pen as I wrote out what I knew was the next right step.

Come back to what you know.

And what I know is the this: *The Self-Trust Model* is powerful.

I've seen the transformations that are possible when you apply it to your life. Even though the specific trust I have in myself to create viral videos is non-existent, the trust I have in the model - hasn't wavered.

As you'll come to see throughout this book, *The Self-Trust Model* can be applied to any area of life. Dating, career, health, finances, spirituality, parenting, personal growth, and the not-for-the-faint-of-heart journey of entrepreneurship.

That being said... I've got a crazy idea...

**What if I applied the model directly to my new struggling business?**

**What if I decided to write about the process, in real time?**

**And, what if I brought you along for the ride?**

Because, what better way to learn something than to watch someone else do it? While also watching them trip and face plant, get back up again, get blindsided, and then attempt to apply the lessons learned.

We'll cover all the basics of *The Self-Trust Model*. I'll share how **ancient wisdom** is deeply ingrained into this framework and I'll also give you the tools you'll need in this **modern world** to actually implement the concepts and practices.

Each time you close this book, I hope you'll feel empowered to apply the model to whatever area of your life is calling for it most right now, and **unlock the wise woman within**.

Hold on, because things are about to get meta. And I honestly have no idea how it's all going to turn out.

# [ 3 ]
# THE SELF-TRUST COMPASS

Before we begin this journey together, I want to give you a sneak peak at *The Self-Trust Compass* - our guide for this adventure and the core of *The Self-Trust Model*™. We'll visit every direction many times throughout this book because they are the fundamentals of Self-Trust. Put it in your pocket, and let's get started...

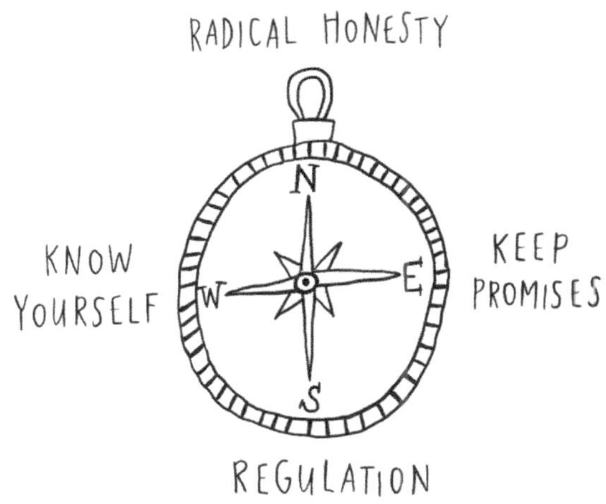

# [ 4 ]
# SEASONS

The structure of this book is broken down into the four seasons of the natural world:

**Spring, Summer, Fall, and Winter.**

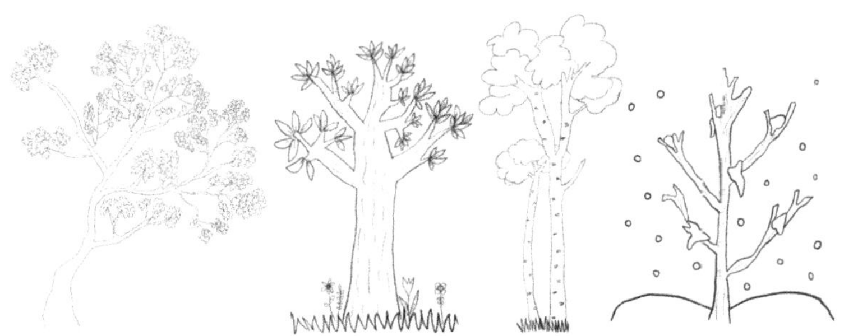

I've learned it's more beneficial (and way more fun) to work *with* nature. Instead of constantly trying to fight against her infinite wisdom.

*Mainly because... she'll always win.* But also, because this perspective can help support your Self-Trust journey.

Connecting with these seasonal rhythms is ancient wisdom that our modern world has disconnected many of us from. The seasons connect us to the cyclical beings we all are - especially as women. We're in a constant state of evolution and change. The seasons remind us that there is value to each stage we're in.

When you can recognize the importance of seasons in the external world, you can also begin to trust yourself to flow with the natural rhythms of creativity and rest. Instead of forcing year-round productivity.

There is a different gift to be found in the darkness of winter than in the light of summer. Trying to be the same every day goes against nature's will. When you're able to understand and honor the season you're in, you're able to leverage the unique magic that each season can offer.

Nature doesn't rush, and yet everything gets done. Sometimes, trust means allowing things to unfold in their own timing. *Including you.*

Trusting yourself isn't about controlling every outcome. By witnessing how nature constantly shifts yet remains whole, you learn to navigate your own life transitions with less fear and more trust in your adaptability.

The seasonal perspective also equips you to honor the transitional spaces *between* the seasons. The solstices and the equinoxes. The portals to the liminal. The bardos.

A beginning and an ending - budded up against each other.

Nature reminds us to bring ritual and ceremony to these moments. And to have reverence for the death and rebirth of who we think we are - many times over.

# [ PART 1 ]
# SPRING

We begin... with the energy of the **Spring Equinox.**

A rebirth.

A peeking out after the dark hibernation of Winter.

A fresh start.

A time to plant seeds.

A gasping moment of awe at sight of the first cherry blossom and being reminded of the fleeting nature of life.

A welcoming of the sun rays.

A life renewed.

Setting the stage for the work we'll do together...

The 'Prologue' & 'Introduction' parts of a book...

Words are defined, intentions are set...

. . .

And we embark on our adventure.

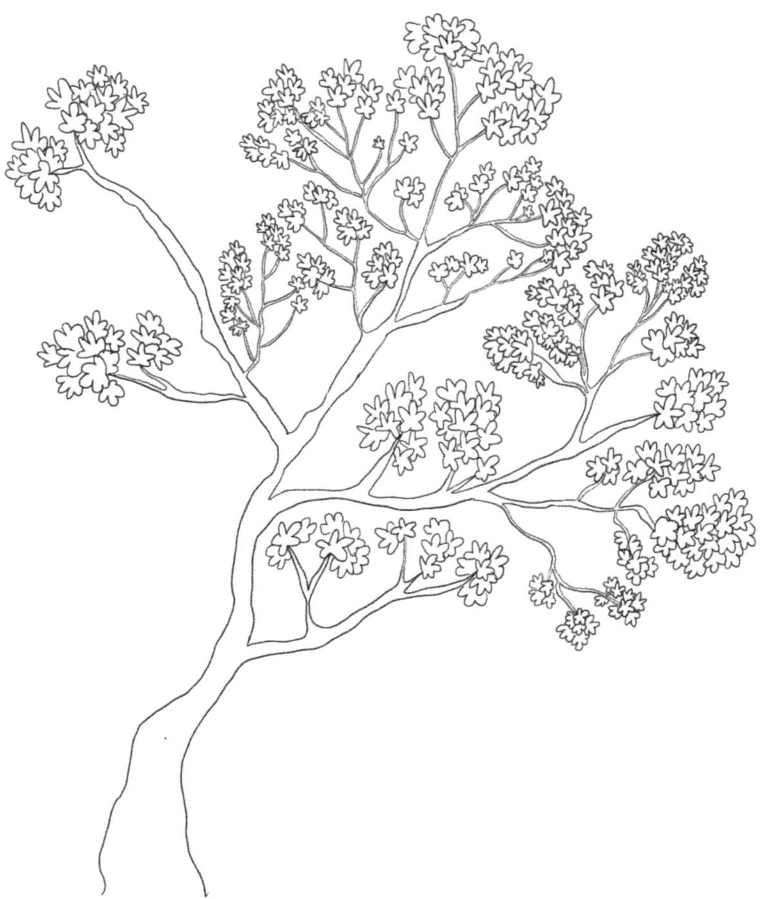

# [ 1 ]
# GIVE ME A SIGN! BUT DON'T TELL ME WHAT TO DO

When I first began my journey to trusting myself again, I didn't know that's what I was doing. I didn't have a framework to follow. I didn't have a mentor or guide. All I knew is I was exhausted from living in a constant state of indecision and insecurity.

Constantly second guessing decisions...

Always doubting myself...

And turning over my power to something outside of me.

**When you're lacking Self-Trust, it can be really tempting to outsource your power to something or someone else**. Then, you don't have to take responsibility for your decisions. Since you didn't *really* make the decision, you can't possibly be to blame when things go poorly, right?

For me, it was "The Universe". In my teens and early twenties, I wanted "Mama U" to step in and make my decisions for me, so I didn't have to. **Give me all the signs!**

For others, it's a doctor, a partner, a teacher, a parent, a friend, a therapist, or a famous self-help author, that they're tempted to give their power to.

However, as much as I wanted the universe to show me a sign or place the exact book in front of me with a clear message when I needed it most, **I don't actually like being told what to do.**

Which is partially why my relationship to the "self-help" section of the bookstore is... complicated.

I especially don't like being told what to do by someone claiming to have a universal answer for everyone. Or a one-size-fits-all prescription from a self-proclaimed guru. Self-help books have never been my jam.

I much prefer dark, gritty, and vulnerable memoirs. I love to hear people's stories. Then, I can pull out the "lessons" from their experiences that resonate with me. I yearn to have spaciousness for my own interpretations.

So where was *that* book when I needed it? The beacon of light when everything felt dark. The guide who'd made it to the other side and lived to tell about it, yet wasn't dogmatic that her path was the only way.

**Where was the self-help book that didn't just tell me what to do?**

# [ 2 ]
# THE ART & SCIENCE OF TRUSTING YOUR INTUITION

To say the last chapter another way...

**I'm not going to tell you how to live your life.**

I am, however, going to make what I think is a *very* strong case for why Self-Trust could be the golden skeleton key to unlock the life you desire.

And the case I'll make to you throughout this book falls at the intersections of:

- "Evidence-Based" and "Woo-Woo"
- "Science" and "Spiritual"
- "Known" and "Unknown"
- "Seen" and "Unseen"
- "Research" and "Mystical"

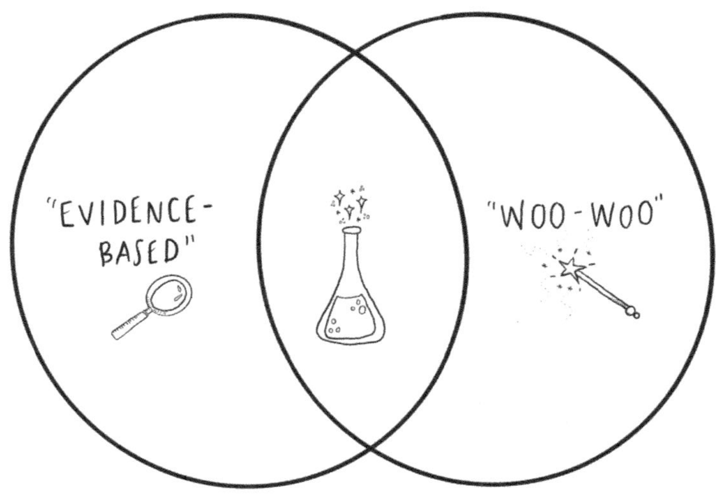


**"Evidence-Based":** Between graduate school, continuing education, advanced specialized training, and my time as a somatic trauma therapist, I've devoted well over 16 years of my life to learning about neuroscience, the nervous system, and how healing *actually* works. I was trained in:

- Somatic Experiencing® (SE)
- Internal Family Systems® (IFS)
- Psychedelic Therapy
- Eye Movement Desensitization & Reprocessing® (EMDR)
- Trauma Focused Cognitive Behavioral Therapy® (TF-CBT)
- Dialectical Behavior Therapy® (DBT)
- Play Therapy
- Sandtray Therapy
- Trauma-Conscious Yoga Method℠
- Trauma Sensitive Yoga
- 200hr Yoga Teacher Training

**These trainings and experiences have absolutely shaped the way I view the human experience and our capacity for change.**

Some of the psychological theories and therapeutic modalities I share in this book have claims backed by a depth of research you can find from the many studies done, especially in the spaces of nervous system healing, EMDR, yoga, IFS, and psychedelic therapy.

However, I'm not claiming the science I'll share in this book is Science with a capital S. Or Truth with a capital T. In general, the word "science" is being used more broadly with less universal consensus on what the definition actually is.

I don't have peer-reviewed studies on Self-Trust to offer you. This isn't a textbook. It's for the introspective lay person.

Additionally, I want to encourage you to take a curious perspective to anything being told to you is "science" or "evidence". If what you're being told is "The Truth", but it goes against what you've experienced to be true or what you're actively seeing in front of you, please don't turn over your power in the name of "Science".

Plus, not all research should be treated equal. And it's always changing.

**"Woo-Woo":** Four years ago, I experienced a *before/after* kind of loss. The kind of loss that radically rearranges your life. When who you were *before* is completely different than who you are *after*. Until you've personally experienced a dark night of the soul, it can be hard to understand how it will fundamentally change you.

Sometimes, traumatic loss allows the veil between our human reality and the "other side" to thin, letting non-ordinary experiences become the new normal. And sometimes, it completely rips the veil to shreds, leaving you spinning in an abyss, questioning everything you've ever known, isolated from reality, and grasping for more. I experienced the latter. **And this also shaped the way I view the human experience and our capacity for change.**

Grief wasn't my first portal into the mystical. I'd long dabbled, sometimes skeptically and sometimes enthusiastically, in what people might consider the "woo-woo" spaces of chakra healing, Traditional Chinese Medicine, acupuncture, Reiki, sound baths, kundalini yoga, energy work, meditation, and tarot. Loss was just the catalyst to lean even deeper in with past life regression, mediums, tantra, and opening myself to synchronicities that impact my decisions.

---

The work that I do with women exists at these intersections. Blending both has been crucial in my own experiences of trying to understand the human experience. It's been about stepping out of the belief that these two worlds are mutually exclusive.

**The book I want to write - includes both.**

[ 3 ]

# A GOLDEN SKELETON KEY

A skeleton key is a type of master key. A key that doesn't just access one door or lock - but is able to unlock many different doors.

So instead of coming to therapy trying to find a key for "confidence" and a key for "better boundaries" and a key for "more self-care" and a key for "healing from trauma" and a key for "overcoming anxiety" – you just need to get this one key.

**The Self-Trust key...**

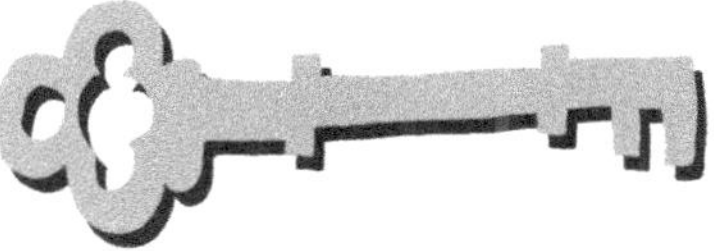

The most profound healing I witnessed during my time as a therapist came on the other side of people learning that they could trust themselves.

**Cultivating more Self-Trust was the catalyst for some of the most beautiful and genuine transformations I ever saw.**

Now, this shouldn't have been a surprise to me. In many ways, it mirrored my own journey. I spent decades feeling deeply insecure, over-thinking and over-explaining myself. It felt safer to outsource my decisions to the universe. I was exhausted from the constant internal tug of war. Stuck in the life-force draining space of indecision. And my physical body was the one paying the price. I tried *everything* to feel more confident and at home in my body.

But it wasn't until I began to deeply trust myself that I experienced genuine and true confidence. And then, I watched as the same thing happened with the women I worked with. It wasn't a "fake-it-till-you-make-it" kind of confidence though. It was a kind of "quiet" confidence that emerged from within. And it was palpable.

> **True confidence doesn't come from knowing exactly what comes next.**
>
> **True confidence comes from knowing you'll be okay - *no matter* what comes next.**

Don't believe me?

Let's look at the origin of the word confidence. *People have understood this connection for centuries.*

*Confidence* stems from the Latin word, *confīdentia*, which translates to... **"Firm Trust"**.

. . .

Here are a few other really cool things we noticed that also came with more Self-Trust:

- A deeper connection to Self and others
- More energy for life
- Clarity about purpose, values, and priorities
- No longer needing a permission slip from someone else to live your life
- Discernment skills & ability to make decisions with confidence
- Ability to give & receive with abundance
- Living an intentional life
- **And... Giving a lot less fucks**

Cultivating more Self-Trust may seem like magic, but it isn't a pill. It's not as easy as the platitude, *"Just trust yourself!"* makes it sound. But once you realize all the doors this key can unlock – it is definitely worth the effort it takes to get it.

When you trust yourself more, you don't have to outsource all your decisions. When you trust yourself, there is a deep knowing that you can handle whatever life throws at you so you don't have to be in a constant state of worry.

**Self-Trust is the antidote to anxiety.**

And even when you make mistakes or things don't go according to plan, the core trust you have in yourself doesn't waver. You begin to see how "mistakes" can actually be a way to build *more* trust in yourself.

This approach paid off in my work as a therapist. Even though we weren't laser focused on "building confidence" or "feeling worthy" or "getting rid of imposter syndrome" - the people I was working with still got what they came for.

*The Self-Trust Model*™ provided structure for them to begin to gradually and consistently build trust in themselves. And as the Self-Trust grew, they noticed they were getting closer to the original goals that had brought them in, in the first place.

They were feeling less anxious and better able to handle stressful situations. Their relationships improved. They were less consumed by their past. They were more confident with their boundaries and life decisions.

And then, they did what I did once I looked down and realized what I was actually holding in my hands... they looked around and began to wonder...

**What other doors will this unlock?**

# [ 4 ]
# NO MORE WHACK-A-MOLE

With this approach, you don't have to play whack-a-mole with every concern, symptom, or crisis of the week. Let me show you what I mean...

Here are some phrases I heard from people in our first session about the reason they were coming to therapy:

- "I'm anxious all the time and can't stop it."
- "I feel out of control."
- "I keep picking the same partner."
- "There's stuff from my past I know I need to deal with."
- "I can't get anything done. I'm always procrastinating."
- "I know I need to set better boundaries, but I don't know how."
- "I can't sleep, my brain never shuts off."
- "I don't know what to do - should I stay or should I go?"
- "I don't know how to deal with all of this stress."

- "I was told I need trauma therapy."
- "I feel like an imposter at work."
- "I'm heartbroken and I don't know how to make it stop."
- "I'm exhausted from trying to be everything to everyone."
- "I feel like I'm just wasting my life away, I don't know what I want to do."
- "My husband said he'd leave me if I didn't fix this."
- "I'm ashamed to talk to anyone else about this."
- **"I don't know why I'm here, but *something* needs to change."**

On the surface, these might all sound pretty different. Someone might even assume they are unrelated to each other. But as we dug deeper, we started to notice the fears living underneath the initial pain points. And they sounded like this:

- Fear of making the "wrong" choice.
- Fear of being misunderstood.
- Fear of being seen.
- Fear of vulnerability + intimacy.
- Fear of losing my mind.
- Fear of rejection.
- Fear of receiving.
- Fear of abandonment.
- **Fear of death.**

Once we identified the core fears living underneath the "reason", we could get curious about the fear. We'd invite the fear to tea. (*This is one of my favorite practices in this model, I'll make sure to tell you about it later.*) And when that fear felt safe enough, it could reveal a belief it was holding onto, often subconsciously:

- Belief that I'm not good enough.
- Belief that I'm not worthy.
- Belief that I'm not loveable.
- **Belief that I can't survive.**

And underneath that belief was an unmet need of trust:

- I don't trust myself to be okay if I make the "wrong" choice.
- I don't trust myself to be okay if this person leaves me.
- I don't trust myself to be responsible with money.
- I don't trust myself to be a good parent.
- I don't trust myself to follow through on what I say I will do.
- I don't trust myself to hold my boundaries.
- I don't trust myself to be okay if people misunderstand me.

Full stop:

- **I don't trust myself.**

## [ 5 ]

# SIGNS YOU MIGHT LACK SELF-TRUST

How do you know if you need to search for the golden skeleton key? Here are a few signs it might be worth it:

- You find yourself stuck in decision paralysis.
- You only seek answers outside yourself.
- You fear making the "wrong" choice.
- You constantly overthink and second guess your decisions.
- You're in people-pleasing mode most of the time.
- You feel bogged down with insecurities.
- You survey 12 people for their opinion each time you have a decision to make.
- You try to control everything.

[ 6 ]

# GOODBYE THERAPY

March 19th

A week ago, I had my final session as a therapist. My final moment of being a space-holder in that way.

I'm shocked at how much relief I feel. It's almost like my intuition knew what she as doing six months ago.

But, I'm sure the existential "Who am I now?!" questioning isn't far away...

I guess "bittersweet" is the cliché, but true way to capture it. I know I'm going to miss my clients and our individual work.

But also... I can't shake how excited I am

for all the groups I'll get to lead now. All my time - freed up for that now.

First up isn't going to be Adventure Club though. The next season of that will have to wait. This one is all online. So, even though I'm taking a big solo trip to celebrate "retirement", I can still run this new group remotely.

My "inner business manager" really likes the idea of this new group. She keeps getting on me about "scaleability" and trying to create a business that makes sense logically.

For her sake, I hope this group can be that.

But if not, I have countless ideas for more groups to run. And now, I no longer have to put them on the back burner because I'm too busy with my therapy practice.

Things are about to look completely different...

# [ 7 ]
# THE REAL THREAT OF INSECURITY

I used to view insecurity as "just" a nuisance. I saw "feeling insecure" about yourself as a limit to your potential, but I didn't think it was existential.

I also convinced myself that my desire to feel more confident was vain and self-centered. With everything else going on in the world, wasn't it selfish of me to want to focus so much energy on wanting to feel more confident?

But I couldn't shake it.

Politely asking the deep insecurity to go away, didn't work. Shaming it also had no lasting effect. And I couldn't seem to find a way to "fake" confidence that withstood any real turbulence.

Every January, when I sat down to write my intentions for the year - it always started the same:

> I Will Feel More Confident in ~~2010~~, ~~2011~~, ~~2012~~, ~~2013~~, ~~2014~~, 2015...

When I was still a baby therapist, I even allowed those thoughts to creep into my work.

*Wouldn't it be a waste of my time to help people focus on building confidence and feeling less insecure? Shouldn't we focus all our work on healing ALL THE TRAUMA - ALL THE TIME?!*

Thankfully, not long into my new career, I realized post-traumatic *growth* was just as valid of an aspiration. My definition of trauma also widened as I learned about *Somatic Experiencing®* and *Internal Family Systems®*.

And I started to help my clients (and myself) see that *these* goals were just as valid:

- To feel confident making decisions.
- To chase my dream of being an artist.
- To live a full and expansive life.
- To learn to trust myself again.
- To enjoy rest and play with my kids.

**I found purpose and meaning in life as I journeyed with others also discovering their purpose and meaning in life.**

---

Recently, I've experienced even more fine tuning regarding my perspectives on insecurity and confidence.

And I think I might have been flat out wrong when I tried to convince myself that feeling insecure wasn't existential.

It actually can be.

As one sometimes does, I recently fell pretty far down a rabbit hole. A cult-documentary rabbit hole that soon illuminated a cult survivor podcast vortex with an infinite supply of episodes highlighting patterns of insecurity.

Once I was able to pop my head back up into reality, I was better able to articulate why focusing my work on healing deep insecurities and building confidence through Self-Trust *is* the hill worth dying on.

Because it *is* that important...

Because nagging insecurity isn't just an annoying itch you wish would go away...

Lacking confidence in yourself isn't just an inner struggle that will hold you back from reaching your potential...

**Deep insecurity in yourself makes you susceptible to danger.**

The more I consumed these post-cult stories, the more this belief was solidified.

And a core theme emerged.

In high-control groups, any trust a person had in themselves was systematically and intentionally eroded through the "teachings", "technology", and under the guise of personal responsibility and human potential.

The bastardization of a few grains of truth.

Trust and good intentions were deliberately weaponized. It appeared that the mission was to disconnect people from their bodies and their inner wisdom.

To dismantle any semblance of Self-Trust.

> Because when you're disconnected from your body and your intuition - ***you become vulnerable.***
>
> Because when you're disconnected from yourself and your inner wisdom - ***you become susceptible to danger.***

This deep insecurity in yourself makes you vulnerable to being taken advantage of. And I'm not only talking about being susceptible to joining a cult. It's the everyday dangers you become vulnerable to being taken advantage of...

- In romantic relationships
- In your career
- In friendships
- In parenting
- In navigating your health
- In choosing a personal growth program
- In watching the news

*The Self-Trust Model*™ has the anti-virus built in.

As we go deeper into this model, you'll see that it intentionally guides you back to yourself. Over and over again.

Back to *your* wisdom.

Back to *your* discernment.

Back to *your* power.

There is no guru. No one with your answers.

I hope through this process, Self-Trust becomes not only your golden skeleton key, but also, your shield if the world around you becomes dangerous.

# [ 8 ]
# DISCOVERING THE MODEL

T*he Self-Trust Model*™ exists because even though most people weren't coming into their first therapy session shouting, *"I just need to trust myself more and everything else will work itself out!"*, that's what was at the heart of it all.

**When Self-Trust grows, everything downstream changes.**

I began noticing patterns and compiling stories. I gathered anecdotal research and I kept track of the practices, exercises, and concepts I repeatedly shared with clients to guide them in trusting themselves more. I noticed where people got stuck (repeatedly) and what helped mobilize them again.

I found myself saying the same things over and over again. And I figured there had to be a way to make this easier on everyone. So while the model didn't come to me all at once, I kept distilling down what I was seeing and what was working.

Modifying and tweaking as we went along.

This first season of *Adventure Club* was the ultimate catalyst to organize everything. And in preparation for our first gathering, I discovered a "hidden" document on my computer that I'd created years before. A place where an earlier version of me had apparently also been keeping track of how to actually cultivate more Self-Trust. She had fundamental aspects of the model written out and didn't even realize it.

As my refinement process continued, something really cool emerged. I discovered one of the biggest selling points of the model:

**This approach allows the source of agency to come from within.**

Because, the specific kind of confidence that comes from more Self-Trust, isn't contingent on the world being any certain way. *Thank god, because the world is hard to keep up with sometimes.*

It's not a one-off solution either. When you do the work to build Self-Trust, you create a solid foundation. It generalizes to other areas of your life. This approach prepares you for the next time that life inevitably throws "life" at you. Because it's going to happen. To you, to me. That's what it means to be human.

Jobs come and go. Babies don't sleep through the night. Friendships evolve. Health isn't guaranteed. Election years happen. People die.

*Life happens.*

Sometimes, it's magical. Sometimes, it's heartbreaking. And oftentimes, it's both.

But when you have a strong sense of trust in yourself, you no longer need to try and control everything around you. Instead, you get to show up in your life, and actually, live.

So, while I understand that applying this model isn't always easy, it can be profound.

And for the people who aren't afraid of a little hard work, exponential growth is possible.

**The juice is definitely worth the squeeze.**

# [ 9 ]
# CONVERGENCE

The *Self-Trust Model™* exists at the convergence of somatic therapy, "parts work", and psychedelic therapy (with or without medicine). Working with the nervous system and all the different "parts" of our psyche is fundamentally baked into how I work with people and think about life. You'll hear me use the language from the specific modalities I was trained in - *Somatic Experiencing®* (SE) *and Internal Family Systems®* (IFS). But you might have other ways of saying the same thing based on your perspectives, trainings, and life experiences. *That's perfect.*

These three highly effective therapeutic approaches are the framework for how I think about healing and, more importantly, *thriving* in life. As you read about *The Self-Trust Model*, sometimes it will be obvious where these modalities have influenced my perspective. But, you may also notice moments when it's more covert. That's how some of our parts and our nervous system likes to operate.

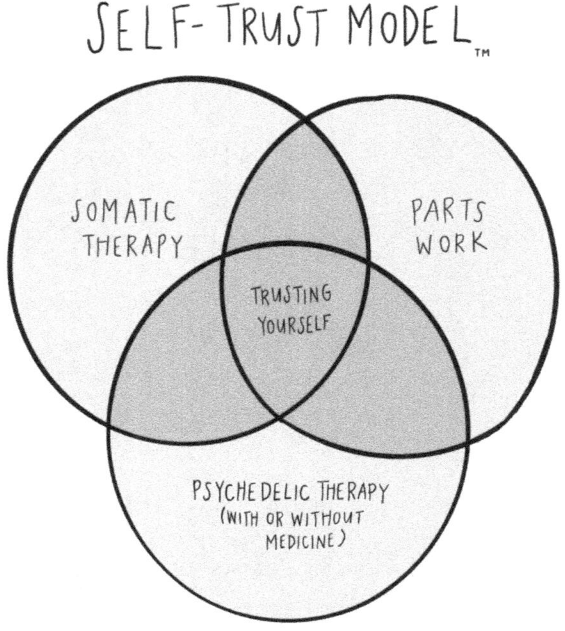


If you notice yourself feeling drawn to any of these modalities, I highly recommend going deeper into each of the original frameworks. While also knowing that what I just described as the "original" frameworks, have their roots in wisdom even deeper. Much deeper. They have roots in ancient wisdom that cultures all over the world have "discovered" in different ways and at different times. Keep digging if you feel called to. Follow your curiosities.

The scope of this book isn't a history lesson to get to the "beginning" of where the wisdom originated. Or a detailed description of each modality. My intention is to make these rediscovered learnings accessible, with the least amount of jargon as possible. I want to offer a concise and structured way to approach living that empowers you to apply the ancient wisdom to your modern, day-to-day life.

# [ 10 ]
# INTEGRATION STARTS WITH PREPARATION

Throughout this book, we're going to talk a lot about how to integrate these practices more fully into your life. Taking them from a concept you read about, to actually allowing them to impact how you show up in relationships, and in your day to day life, for the better. Because you can have all the profound mystical experiences and spiritual awakenings you want, but if you're still running away from your life every chance you get - *what's the point?*

**The best integration starts with preparation.**

How you prepare for an experience not only has a huge impact on the experience itself, but also on how well you'll be able to integrate it later on.

So, let's talk about mystical experiences for a bit. This is a common way to describe what can happen during an intentional psychedelic or plant medicine experience.

> "Psychedelic" means mind-revealing or soul-manifesting.

> Psychedelics expand awareness and amplify... everything. *Especially things you've been trying to avoid.*

You can enter into a non-ordinary state of consciousness (NOSC) through ingesting a psychedelic compound. The "mystical experience" that can follow is characterized by:

- a sense of unity and oneness
- feelings of awe and ecstasy
- ineffability (inability to describe it in words)
- the transcendence of time and space

Although, when I think of the last bullet point, I'm reminded of my psychedelic therapy training and the words I heard from *Christopher Bache:*

> *"Find balance between transcending time & space and being grounded in time & space."*

His advice came after 73 therapeutically structured, high-dose LSD sessions over 20 years. In this instance, I'm really going to try to apply the lessons he learned without having to experience it for myself.

You can read more of the lessons he learned from those experiences in his book, *LSD And the Mind of the Universe.*

---

It's also very likely that if I was introduced to psychedelics in my early twenties, I wouldn't have been able to find the balance he's referring to. I likely would've recklessly been using the medicine. They would've been another form of escapism.

Another way for me to leave my body. But a way that I could portray as "healing".

I'm grateful to have discovered the healing potential of psychedelics after over a decade of deep inner healing that *didn't* involve plant medicines. And, *after* I relearned what it was like to embody my body.

My experience would've likely been very different if our paths had crossed earlier. That's why I don't subscribe to the idea that plant medicines and psychedelics are universally good for everyone. There are *many* caveats.

---

For the sake of this book, we're not just talking about eating magic mushrooms, drinking Ayahuasca in the jungle, participating in Ketamine Assisted Psychotherapy (KAP), or having 70+ acid trips.

There are many ways to experience different states of consciousness without medicine. We enter a different state of consciousness every night when we dream. We can intentionally access a different state through breathwork, meditation, sex, and even dancing to music.

**Want a really profound experience to meet the Divine?**

Sit in silence under a tree for 24 hours. Without your phone.

Seriously... try it.

All this to say, psychedelic experiences in the way you might be thinking are *not* a requirement to work with the *principles* of psychedelic therapy. You don't have to ingest anything to experience the powerful healing that's possible.

And honesty, not everyone should.

Before you embark on any type of potentially life-altering experience, it can be incredibly beneficial to prepare yourself physically, mentally, emotionally, spiritually, relationally, and logistically. Bringing ceremony and ritual to working with different states of consciousness can amplify their effectiveness. And it can be helpful to start with the end in mind.

The preparation principles we'll explore can be applied to any new beginning or experience you have. You can go through this process before you go on a yoga retreat, before you begin therapy, in preparation for childbirth, as you begin dating again, or before you read the rest of this book.

**Preparation Principles:**

- Set
- Setting
- Dose

[ 11 ]

# SET

Set refers to your mindset or mental state. This is where intention setting comes in. An opportunity to get clear about the aspirations you have for the experience. *What is the energy you want to bring and what are you open to receive?*

Reflection questions can be a great way for intentions to reveal themselves to you:

- What regrets or resentments am I ready to let go of?
- What self-limiting beliefs am I holding onto?
- What is my relationship with stillness?
- Where do I feel most lit up in life?
- Teach me about [love/forgiveness/trust].
- Show me [my fears/possibility/joy].
- Where am I waiting for permission?

Setting an intention for an experience is different than having an agenda for it. If you have an agenda for exactly how something needs to go, there's a good chance you're not operating from your wise and competent "Adult Self". You're likely operating from a different "part" of you.

It's the difference between setting out with a bow, arrows, and a hunter mentality that you won't return home until you've killed exactly what you need. Or setting out with a basket and an open heart to gather whatever you happen to find.

A powerful reminder before you do any type of challenging personal growth work is this:

- When something beautiful or magical emerges, **move towards it**, connect with it, and allow yourself to surrender into it.
- When something challenging, scary, confusing, or disturbing emerges, **move towards it** with curiosity and inquiry.

Things aren't necessarily "good" or "bad". They just are. And when we go towards them with curiosity, we can learn so much about ourselves.

Intention setting is a fundamental part of the group work I do when we're working with *The Self-Trust Model*. Which is why I created the *Reflect + Set* guide. It's a 20-page booklet to help you reflect on the past six months and then guide you to set intentions for the upcoming six months.

When I decided to apply *The Self-Trust Model* to my new business endeavor, I knew this is where I needed to start. Taking time to reflect on life and set intentions for the future is a non-negotiable if I want to live an intentional life. And have an intentional business.

I know how powerful a practice like this can be. It's not new to me. But somehow I was still surprised when I sat down and actually did it. Reviewing the past six months was further confirmation of how much I've been working. Honestly, part of me felt proud as I wrote all of what had happened in the first six months of the year. While another part of me asked, *"Dude, what's it going to take for you to slow down?"*

Something kind of monumental happened that I'd forgotten about until this exercise. I let my therapy license expire. *Well, at least one of the three states I was licensed in.* It was up for renewal at the same time as my practice was ending. I considered scrambling to finish their specific requirements, fill out paperwork, and pay hundreds of dollars to have, what? A safety net in case I failed and needed to go back to being a therapist?

I considered renewing the license, buying myself two more years. Bargaining a bit with myself by reminding myself what all I had to do to *get* the license. Was it really worth it to just let it all go away with the 'delete' of an email?

But I know the part of me who was trying to bargain. Trying to logic her way out of fear. Trying to avoid doing the thing she knew was right. I know her well now. She makes a lot of sense to me. I have a lot of compassion for her.

And also - she's no longer in charge of making my decisions.

---

Taking time to reflect opens up space for deeper intention setting. Beyond the surface level goals. When I think about my intention for the next phase of creating my new business, I come back to my values and the life I truly want to live.

Because my intentions are both about what I want to create and put out into the world for others and also the life I want to create for myself and my family.

**I want to continue creating containers for intimate groups of women to come together and do cool shit.** I want to create spaces where we can talk about the taboo and what lurks in the shadows. Where we can make mistakes and repair wholeheartedly. Where we can contradict ourselves and disagree with each other. Where we use the word 'fuck' generously and in all it's contexts. I want to witness moments of true vulnerability and connection. I want to learn from every woman in the circle with me. I want to experience the full spectrum of the human experience together. I want our laughter and our tears to morph into one. I want to sit in the questions of our existence. And then come up for air and talk about a new silly trending video. I want to offer this transformative space to women who also desire this kind of soul-connection. And I want to do it over never-ending, sacred cups of tea.

**I also want to write things that make people feel *big* things.** I want to write in ways that allow people to feel seen. I want to offer these things, because other women have offered them to me. And I understand, on a deep cellular level, how priceless these gifts are.

I want to "do" all of that. And, I also want to get to know the part of me that doesn't have to work so hard, all the time. I want the part of me that thinks hard work = value, to get a break for a while. I want to learn to rest. And then, I want to learn to *enjoy* resting. I want to work with my cycles. Allowing bursts of creative energy to come through without shame for working "too much" and then hold the rest periods with reverence.

I want to be outside hiking - everyday. I want to spend quality time with our girls. I want to have weekly body work sessions to nurture this vessel. I want to buy the organic food we want without thinking about the price. I want to go on epic adventures with my family and friends.

And, maybe most importantly, I want to not feel guilty in my desire for this life of "more" I crave.

---

A final note on intention setting from the perspective of the guide and the one holding space... either for a medicine journey or the journey this book will take you on:

The intention I learned to embody as I held space for someone else was referred to as the **"Grandmother Approach":**

- Crossed-legged on the floor, arms out, palms up.
- The energy and mantra of: *"I'm here. And you got this."*

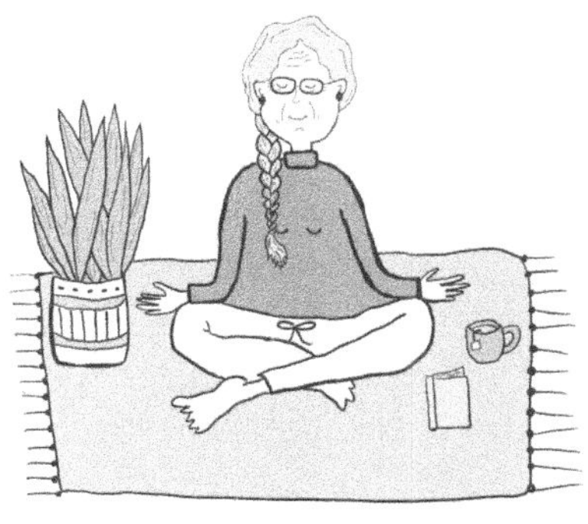

I'd love to remind you of that right now. Before we go any further.

I'm here. The model to guide you is here. Others who have done this work are here. And, ultimately...

**You fucking got this.**

# [ 12 ]
# SETTING

Setting refers to your physical surroundings. It could be a spiritual retreat center, a therapist's office, at home, or at a rave. The environment you take mushrooms in has a huge impact on the experience you'll have. It's the difference between having a "bad trip" surrounded by hundreds of strangers at a festival or entering into difficult material in your psyche with a trusted guide to help you through it.

Settings aren't "bad" or "good". It's remembering your intention and then choosing a setting that supports the intention.

Things to consider when you choose your setting for a psychedelic experience:

- Do you want to be inside or outside?
- Can you limit distractions? (Ex. clean house beforehand, turn off phone)
- Access to a bathroom.
- Who do you want to be with you?
- How can you align the setting with your intention?

- Consider music, lighting, and ambiance.
- Ability to adjust your setting as you go.
- Consider having access to a pen and notebook.

---

You can apply the psychedelic therapy principles of setting, to doing the work inside this book as well. Remember, applying these concepts doesn't require you to take any drugs.

You can still align your setting with your intentions for this work.

A lot of "the work" you'll do to build Self-Trust requires you to go out into the world and live your life. This isn't the type of change that can solely occur in a therapist's office or a corner nook of your room.

*And.* I still encourage you to create a physical space to represent where you do this work. It's the place you read this book. It's where you connect to yourself. It's where you reflect. It's where you do the exercises. It's where you breathe. It's where you write. It's where you move. It's where you remember *who the fuck you are.*

It's a physical space that holds the energy of the intentions you hold in your heart.

This doesn't mean you can't go into the forest alone or take this book on a plane ride. Please do that too. But this is about creating a physical anchor point to return to. It's a tangible and visual reminder of your intention and the work you're doing. It's about creating an intentional space to connect with yourself as you navigate this journey.

For over a decade, my "setting" has been an altar in my home. A short table that could hold my journals, the books I was reading, trinkets from my travels, vision boards, pictures of loved ones, and lots of tea. For me, this isn't religious, but it can be if that's what works for you. It's my physical reminder to slow down and connect to myself.

During my nomadic years, I had a "traveling altar". A small wicker basket that could hold everything and then be turned upside down to act as the table once I landed in my new temporary home. A tether when my only constant was... change.

Don't overthink it. It can be a corner of your room, a window seal, a spot on your couch with an end table, or your bathroom counter. Make it work for you. And let it evolve with you.

**Ideas for creating an alter or intentional space in your home:**

- Things gathered from nature
- Travel trinkets + treasures
- Photos
- Writing supplies
- Candles
- Books
- Things that remind you of loved ones
- Artwork + crafts
- Representations of the things you want in life
- Incense
- Things to represent the seasons
- Salt Lamp
- Reminders of your ancestors
- Rocks + crystals
- Fresh flowers
- Jewelry

# [ 13 ]
# DOSE

Dose refers to how much of the substance (*psilocybin, ketamine, LSD, etc*) you ingest. There are people who swear by microdosing (taking a very small amount that is below the threshold of perception). Those who believe you need to take a "heroic dose" to have the most healing journey. And then there are the people who believe dose doesn't actually matter that much and you'll always have the experience you're meant to have, regardless of how much you take.

A good place to begin when you're thinking about dose, is how to align your dose with your intention. As well as your past experience with the particular substance.

**Common advice if it's your first time taking a psychedelic is to start *low and slow*.**

As a somatic therapist, this approach always resonated. It's conducive to the way the nervous system operates best. Some of the critics of psychedelic assisted psychotherapy center around the cathartic nature of the experience. It's asserted that one high-dose psychedelic journey is the equivalent of ten years of traditional talk therapy.

Tempting, right?

Especially for those of us with a sense of urgency or proclivity for bypassing.

But what that assertion doesn't often include, is the years of integration often needed for the psychedelic journey to actually be incorporated into your life and relationships.

---

Anything that is perceived as "too much", "too soon", or "too fast" can be registered as a threat in our nervous system.

This is where titration comes in.

**Titration = little bits at a time.**

It's a word that *Somatic Experiencing* borrowed from chemistry.

Imagine you have one beaker with Liquid Compound #1 and another beaker with Liquid Compound #2. Depending on what the compounds are, but for the sake of this visual, if you pour Compound #1 quickly into Compound #2, the entire beaker blows up in your face.

It's too much. Too fast.

Titration is the slow addition of Compound #1 into Compound #2. Adding one tiny drip at a time. By going slow and allowing time to settle in between drips, you can combine the full amount of both compounds.

Without having to call the fire department.

Titration can be an essential element of success when you approach making changes in your life.

Remember:

- You don't have to do everything all at once.
- You don't have to seek big, cathartic releases to have long-lasting change.

**Slowly, is the fastest way to heal.**

Even when the change you want to make is a "good thing", your nervous system can still register it as a threat because it's unfamiliar.

You may have really positive intentions for growth and change. You might be excited to dive headfirst into new healthy habits or amped up to try the latest trending hacks, but if your system registers it as too much, it can still shut down.

Within this approach, I want to encourage you to work WITH your nervous system. Not overwhelm it. Because sustainable change doesn't happen when you're in a state of overwhelm.

---

Now, this is where I encourage you to take in the material slowly.

One chapter = one drip

- Allow space in between the drips.
- Allow the information to actually land in your system, before moving onto the next one.

When you approach this work slowly, you gradually build more and more capacity in your nervous system. And more capacity in your nervous system, is what allows for your innate healing wisdom to emerge.

I encourage you to go slow and listen to your body as you take in this information. Listen to when your body is ready for more. When you feel your body leaning in. When you feel the pull.

**Trust the pull.**

And, pay attention to when your body needs a break. A deeper breath. A slower tempo. A walk in the woods without your phone. When you feel the pause.

**Trust the pause**.

---

Repetition is also helpful. Repetition can be soothing to our brain and nervous system. It can help coax us *out* of a state of overwhelm. We often need to hear things in multiple ways and at different times for it to really sink in.

Reread chapters. Try out the practices multiple times. Give something a second chance, even if you initially hate it.

Remind yourself... there's no rush.

**It takes as long as it takes.**

[ 14 ]

# INCONVENIENT INTUITION

May 3rd

"It takes as long as it takes." ??? Seriously? Who says shit like that?!

How did none of my clients ever punch me in the face when I said that to them?

I actually DO need to figure out what comes next... and fast. I need replace my old income. I need to get these groups up and running.

Not to mention, that at 37, I decided now was the perfect time to come to the realization that I DO want to get pregnant. There's a lot to figure out. This actually IS urgent.

This laundry list of things I've been doing since

I closed my therapy practice, is literally exhausting - even just to look at.

It's no wonder I feel like I'm doing a shit job at a ton of things. Because I kind of am.

But I just keep bargaining with myself. Trying to pretend I'll actually slow down... next week.

When it's convenient, then, I'll pull back.

But I know myself better than that.

And I know that following my intuition only when it's convenient... isn't enough.

And even though I've gotten "better" at listening to my inner whisper before she has to scream at me...

> "Better" does not mean perfect.
> "Better" does not mean always.

She may not be screaming at me just yet, but she's definitely speaking to me in a stern, slightly raised voice. If I don't change my ways soon, she'd surely pull out the "I'm disappointed in you" card. My personal kryptonite.

Fuuuuuuuuuuuuuck.

I think I know what I need to do.

I think I've known for a while now.

I know I can't keep doing things the way I have been. I can't keep doing ALL the things. I need to choose. I need to focus on just one thing - and actually do it well.

Okay great... so why do I keep feeling pulled to the "one thing" being the reflection series I wrote after I closed by practice?

The thing I've been calling "The 13 Lessons"...

There's no way that can make any money. And isn't that the point of my business?

Fuck. I don't know why. But I know that's what I need to do.

Maybe I can do it for just a few months.

Yeah, three months is do-able.

I have to keep running the online group until it's finished, but I won't start anything else.

I'll focus on only "The 13 Lessons" for three months. And if nothing comes of it...

I can always go back to doing all the things, in the fall.

# [ 15 ]
# ANCIENT WISDOM

*I'm sorry.*

*Please forgive me.*

*Thank you.*

*I love you.*

These are the words that came to me during my first high dose mushroom experience. On repeat. Over and over. I said them. Out loud or just in my mind, I have no idea.

*I'm sorry.*

*Please forgive me.*

*Thank you.*

*I love you.*

Then, the order changed...

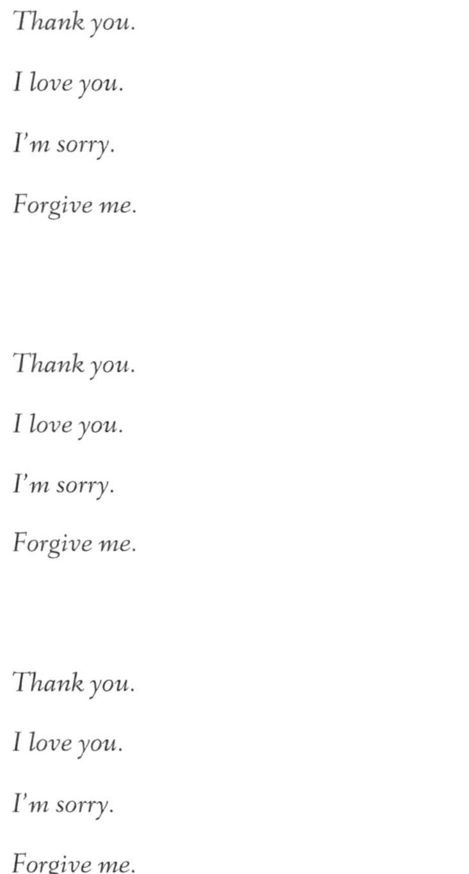

*Thank you.*

*I love you.*

*I'm sorry.*

*Forgive me.*

*Thank you.*

*I love you.*

*I'm sorry.*

*Forgive me.*

*Thank you.*

*I love you.*

*I'm sorry.*

*Forgive me.*

Ahhh yes, this is the order that feels right...

This is the order I wrote on a sheet of paper nearby. Over and over again. At the end of each sentence - adding someone's name. Sometimes adding my own name.

True to "Mama Shroom Time", I have no idea how long I stayed in this repetitive state of gratitude, love, and forgiveness. Probably only a few seconds in real life. But I do know there were pages filled with these words.

Words I assumed came from within me.

Only relevant to me.

***Silly me.***

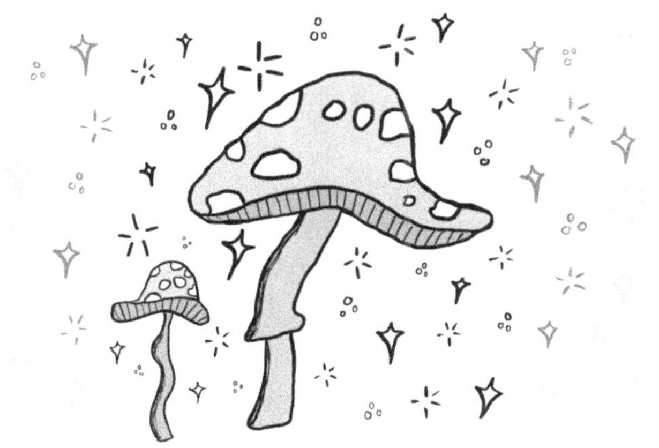

Many months later, in a conversation with another psychedelic therapist - these words from my experience came flooding back to me. I quickly found the journal and read it to her. Reading the phrase as I'd written it.

She looked at me curiously and then asked, *"Have you heard of the Ho'oponopono Prayer?"*

Even though I had no idea what word she'd just said, the answer was easy.

No.

I had no idea what she was asking about.

*"Well, I think you just said it...."* she responds.

And then she does a quick internet search to recite the Hawaiian prayer and its meaning to me. As she continues on with what she knows about this ancient healing and forgiveness practice, I try to not let the tears break the surface of my eyes.

My body was having an intense reaction I couldn't make rational sense of. I continued on, trying to listen to her, knowing my human brain wouldn't be able to keep up with her words.

---

This is just one example of wisdom I thought came to me through my own brain, from my own experiences. But in reality, it is ancient wisdom from an entire culture I don't have any conscious connection to. A prayer I'd never heard of before. A traditional practice I'd never been exposed to. But it came to me - when I needed it the most.

## [ 16 ]

# MODERN OVERWHELM

Earlier, I asserted that sustainable change doesn't happen when you're feeling overwhelmed. And if you're anything like the women I've worked with, feeling overwhelmed is as common as your morning cups of coffee.

Feeling overwhelmed can stem from the pressure to be everything to everyone. To be Superwoman - *all the time.* And underneath that, maybe a desire to *never* disappoint anyone.

**I saw women striving to be the best:**

- Pinterest Mom
- Boss Bitch
- Activist for every cause
- Sexy Partner & Wife always up for something new
- Doting Daughter
- Friend with endless time and patience
- PTA Powerhouse
- Employee of the Month

And - they were also putting immense pressure on themselves to be "good" at self-care. Scrolling social media to hear what the latest "expert" recommends and trying to apply every piece of advice, all at once.

**They were trying to implement all the strategies:**

- Daily meditation
- Acupuncture
- Yoga retreats
- Going to float tanks
- "Resetting" their nervous system
- Mouth taping
- Yoni steaming
- Weekly therapy
- Cold plunging
- 2-hour morning routines
- Red light therapy
- IV drips
- Cutting people out of their life in the name of "boundaries"
- Cryotherapy
- Fasting
- Past Life Regression

If reading these lists feels both overwhelming *and* familiar, I promise you - **you're not alone.**

I've seen thousands of overwhelmed women trying to do "all the things". And here's what I know from a nervous system perspective. When you're feeling *overwhelmed*, it's a good sign that your nervous system is in a ***freeze*** state. It might be a "functional freeze", and you're still able to check things off your to-do list. People looking at you might not even suspect it, but in the nervous system - it's a ***freeze*** state nonetheless.

And just like the fight or flight energy, the freeze state in our nervous system is all about *survival.* None of these survival states place judgment on *how* you survive. They just care about surviving the threat, and you can deal with the consequences of how you survived, later.

But, unlike the pure mobilization energy of fight or flight; freeze is like having both the gas *and* the brake floored.

Just like a car, it's literally exhausting.

You have all the intense survival energy of fight or flight *underneath* the immobilization of the freeze state.

---

Take a moment here... just to pause.

**Check in with your body...**

- Do *you* notice a sense of overwhelm in your body?
- Do you also know what it feels like to try to do "all the things"?
- Is that working for you?

I'll keep reminding you what I've seen (and experienced) over and over again.

**Slowly, is the fastest way to heal.**

Trying to add in a bunch of different healing strategies and practices from a bunch of different voices doesn't help long term. You might get some quick wins, but likely, you'll end up back in a pattern of overwhelm. Spinning your wheels. Doing all the things. You'll get stuck, once again, in what's *not* working.

An alternative to this cycle of modern overwhelm, is doing the work to secure the golden skeleton key we talked about earlier. Because, when you cultivate more trust in yourself, YOU become the expert on your own life. YOU have the confidence and discernment skills to know when to discover the answers inside, and when (*and how*) to seek support externally.

You'll trust yourself to prioritize the roles you play in other people's lives. You'll trust yourself to know which self-care practices actually make sense for you, in *this* season of life.

---

Speaking of the season of life that you're in, I want to remind you of something that part of you may already know.

Not all the practices and exercises that are included in this book are going to resonate for you *right now*. That's okay. In fact, it's *more* than okay.

To be even more transparent, **I *hope* that some of the ideas and tools I share DO NOT resonate in your life right now.** I *hope* that being exposed to some of these practices, connects you to your "No".

Because connecting to your "No" - connects you to your power.

And the connection to inner power can mobilize you to come *out* of overwhelm.

## [ 17 ]
# DEFINITIONS

Wait.

How have we gotten this far into a book about Self-Trust, and I haven't even given you a clear definition?

Maybe you've had a chance to consider your own definition of what it means to trust yourself? I hope so.

Either way, here's mine:

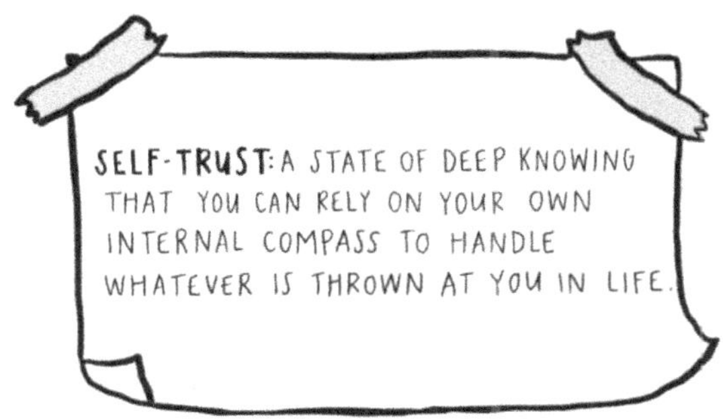

Again, the kind of confidence that comes from more Self-Trust isn't contingent on the world being any certain way. Or treating you any certain way. That's my favorite part about this approach. It's not a one-off solution.

When you do the work to get the golden skeleton key, you can carry it with you, and open any door.

*Is there anything you want to add to the definition?*

[ 18 ]

# YOU ARE HERE

Imagine this Self-Trust journey you're embarking on is actually a physical hike in unfamiliar woods. Having a map could be a great idea; especially for novice hikers.

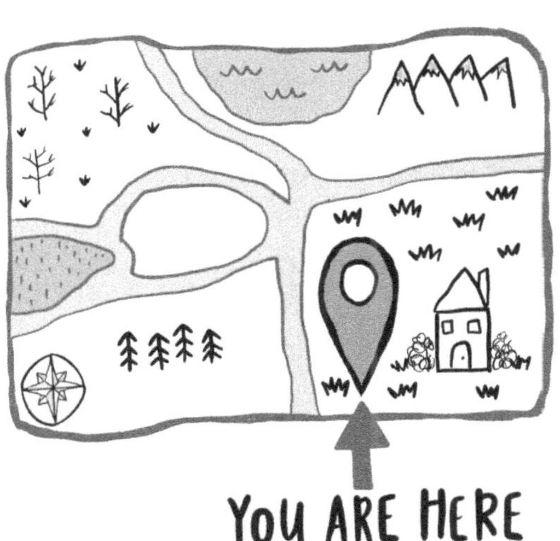

When you're looking at a map, it's really important to begin by identifying your starting point. You'll need to find the 'You Are Here' pin on the map.

Maybe this is the first time you're approaching personal growth and the life goals you have through the Self-Trust perspective. Or maybe you're re-reading this for the 4th time - applying the model to a different area of your life.

Your specific starting point doesn't actually matter. What matters is that you identify it. Accurately. Not what you *wish* your starting point was. But what it actually *is*. Right now, in *this* moment.

Time to get *radically honest* with yourself.

---

First, locate your ***Self-Trust Map + Scale***

Your journey of Self-Trust is going to be unique to you. I can't just give you my map and have you follow my exact steps. Or the steps that other women have taken with this model. My starting point is going to be different from yours. My desired destination may be far away from where you want to end up. This is why you have to really dig deep and get honest with yourself. Because blindly following someone else's map may take you to a place you don't even want to go.

This particular exercise is really helpful for those of you who want something tangible to track. Personal growth can often feel abstract and messy at times. It can be disorienting. And definitely *not* linear. It's often cyclical and seasonal.

Having something concrete to anchor back to throughout the journey can be helpful. Especially on the days it feels like you're not making progress or everything is worse than when it started. ***Pro Tip: Expect to have those days.***

This particular map has space to track your progress, using a 0-10 scale, over six months. Breaking it down with monthly check-ins to track your progress. You can repeat it as many times as is helpful.

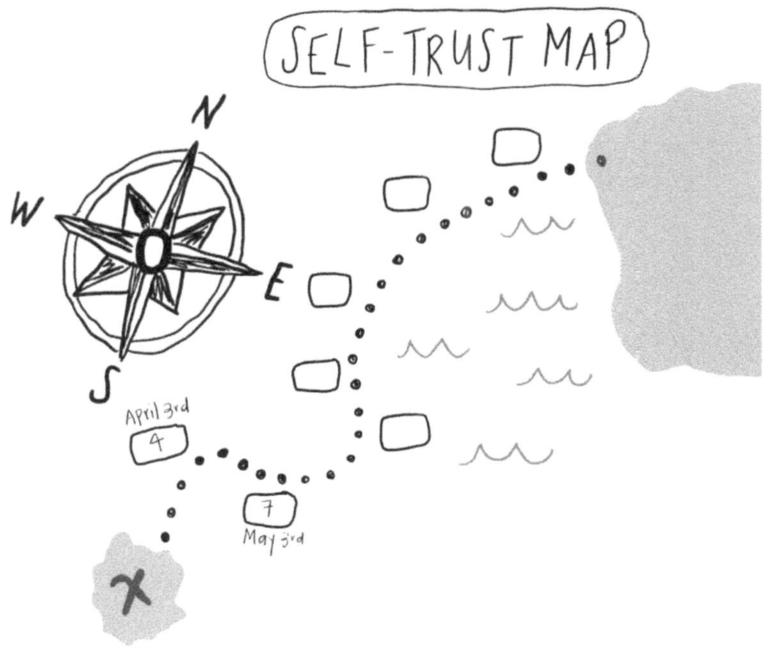


Let's first start by identifying the area of your life you want to track.

I've seen this done 2 ways:

- **General Self-Trust:** How much you trust yourself overall. I often see people who want to look at Self-Trust more generally their first time through the model.
- **Specific Self-Trust:** How much you trust yourself in a specific area of your life. This can be easier to track because it's more specific. Choose one area of life to track and focus on for six months. This is the area of your life you'll want to apply all the exercise and concepts to.
  - Health (mental, emotional, physical, etc)
  - Career
  - Parenting
  - Dating
  - Relationship with money
  - Spiritual practices
  - Ability to make decisions

Once you've decided what you'll be tracking for at least the next six months, ask yourself:

> On a scale of 0-10: How much do I trust myself in__________?

First, I encourage you to close your eyes and just notice if a number initially comes to mind. How does your body immediately respond to the question? Just notice.

Then, when you're ready, let's take a look at the scale so we know what the numbers mean in the context of Self-Trust.

**Let's begin at the bottom with zero:**

**0- Lost in *Life-Scripts***: You automatically follow societal or external *Life-Scripts* without questioning if they align with your true desires or values. You fear making the "wrong choice" and feel trapped in decision paralysis. Insecurities bog you down, preventing you from trusting yourself. You allow (and sometimes invite) others to make decisions for you.

**5- Tentative Decision Maker**: You're breaking free from decision paralysis and insecurities, gradually embracing your inner guidance. While you still experience hesitation and uncertainty, you're starting to use your body as a compass for decision making. You're becoming more aware of your desires and values, allowing them to inform your choices.

**10- Confident + Active Life Participant:** You're confidently engaging in life, taking responsibility for your decisions. Trusting your inner wisdom, you seek answers within yourself before looking for external validation or advice. Connected to your body and intuition, you use discernment and intention to make life choices. You're an active participant in shaping your own life.

---

Now, here's where I tell you how this exercise isn't *just* a practice in identifying a number and tracking the changes.

It's also about tracking the *process* of doing the exercise. When you first asked yourself how much you trust yourself:

- Did a number immediately pop into your mind?
- Did you find yourself bouncing between two numbers?

- Did you have parts trying to "convince" you of a number?
- Did you experience clarity or certainty about the number?

Just allow yourself to notice what the process was like for you, without judging it. As you revisit this exercise at least five more times to fill out the map, I encourage you to track how the number changes. And, also notice how the process of identifying the number evolves too. Both are indicators of how much you trust yourself.

---

Throughout this book, we'll talk about your *Future Self* quite a bit. And I want to encourage you to take a moment to think about her, **right now**. Building a relationship with your past selves and future selves can strengthen the trust you have in yourself in the present moment.

*Consider:*

- How can you support your *Future Self* right now?
- How can you set her up for success?

*One idea:*

If this practice resonated at all with you, I encourage you to set her up for success by scheduling the next five check-ins, *right now*. Don't rely on your memory if you don't have to. Put this book down. Grab your calendar. One month from today, schedule check in#2. You'll go through this exact same process again. Then, schedule the rest of the check in's to fill out this map.

Now that you've got your reminders in your calendar, ask yourself if there's any other way you can be kind to your *Future Self* or set her up for success.

Quiet the external and listen. Maybe she has something to share with you...

## [ 19 ]
# START WITH THE END IN MIND

"The physicality of death destroys us.
But the idea of death saves us."
- Irvin Yalom

Death isn't most people's favorite topic. In fact, many people go to great lengths to avoid talking about it or even acknowledging it. We have a lot of shared platitudes, after someone dies, to distance ourselves from the reality of everyone's inevitable end. We talk *around* death in the name of being "tactful" and "considerate". But it's not *just* the death of our physical body that we collectively try to avoid.

We often try to put blinders on to *all* endings. In the excitement of a new relationship, new job, new school, new city, new self-help program, we don't want to acknowledge the one constant. The truth that everything will change, evolve, and ultimately, end.

Endings can be really scary and painful. They can crack us open in unimaginable ways that we can't ever fathom coming out the other side.

But sometimes, *we're* the ones who make an ending harder than it has to be. By not acknowledging it.

I can't speak for all people in the world who've ever lost a loved one and were promptly offered a *"She's in a better place"* or a *"God needed him more"*, but I've heard from quite a few who are in agreement with just how shitty it feels. How the platitudes make it worse and actually disconnect the grieving person, even more. Compounding more loss on top of overwhelming grief.

**The avoidance and denial is where the suffering thrives.**

It's another reminder of how the things we are most scared of, are often the same things that can liberate us when we acknowledge and accept them.

Death has taught me many things about endings - that don't just apply to death. Death has taught me to strive to have endings that honor what existed.

When you're able to intentionally bring to mind the end, at the beginning - so much of the experience can change. When you're able to be deliberate about an ending, it allows for you to rewrite the script on what endings mean.

You even get to explore what it could look like to do an ending "well".

---

The same is true for this book.

It will end. The practices will come to a close. New concepts will cease to exist. You will close the back cover. Allow yourself to consider...

**Who might you be when you read the final page?**

[ 20 ]

# CONNECTIONS WITH YOUR FUTURE SELF

Have you had a chance to begin connecting with your *Future Self*? Remember, nurturing the relationship you have with her can strengthen your *current* Self-Trust. Here are a few practical ways of supporting this relationship:

- *Future Self Reflections* meditation

- Write letters in your journal from your *Future Self* with words of wisdom and advice.
- Send audio messages to your *Future Self*.

    - Same idea as the handwritten letters, but sent in audio form.
- Do something today your *Future Self* will thank you for.
    - Follow through on a commitment.
    - Opt for sleep over late night scrolling.
    - Say 'No' when your body says 'No'
    - Don't eat the food your body doesn't tolerate well.
    - Have the hard conversation.

Doing something my *Future Self* would thank me for hasn't always been my way of operating in the world. There have been plenty of times in the midst of making a not-so-great decision, I said to myself, "Well, that's *Future Emily's* problem to figure out!"

I used to joke about my "terrible boss" when I'd wake up and see my schedule full of way too many client sessions and no break to eat.

*I was self-employed.*

As I transition away from a career and business structure that was set on auto-pilot, I know I need to do things differently. I know listening to the inner whisper-turned-stern voice is the kindest thing I can do for my *Future Self.*

Which brings me to one final *Future Self* practice. And brings us back to where we left off last chapter...

Death.

**Administer a post-mortem on your goal - at the beginning.**

*Start with the end in mind.*

Visualize: You're at the end of the timeframe you set for your goal. You didn't reach it. You failed. Miserably. Reflect on why your goals were not achieved.

When I did a post-mortem on my new business, I jumped six months ahead to the end of the year. I asked myself:

- Why did everything fail?
- Why is everyone disappointed?
- Why does my to-do list still have hundreds of items?
- Why did I lose trust in myself to run my business?
- Why do I feel less connected to my family and friends?

The consistent answer for all the questions was simple. And annoying.

*I didn't slow down and prioritize.*

The version of me who relies solely on hard-work, doesn't know how to delegate, and thinks she has to replace her old income immediately, had a rough wake up call at the end of the year. She was not at all where she thought she'd be when she decided to close down her therapy practice.

And worst of all? She was also not getting any more quality time with the people she loves or downtime to enjoy life. She was working harder, but not smarter. And she was six months closer to one of the most common deathbed regrets,

*"I wish I hadn't worked so hard".*

Or maybe in 50 years the new #1 regret will be, *"I wish I hadn't spent so much time learning how to promote my business on social media."*

Time will tell.

Let's end this chapter with one of my favorite practices to connect with your *Future Self*. It was first introduced to me by therapist and guide, *Jessica Waclawski*.

Send her a handwritten letter.

Get out your best stationary or scribble in whatever notebook you have closest to you. But sit down and write a letter to the version of you at *the end* of this book.

Let yourself write whatever comes to your mind. You might share about where you're at in life now. You might tell her about where you hope to be over the next few months. You might share a hidden desire you have. Think about her. Write to her. Write whatever flows through your pen.

Don't overthink it.

When you're finished, seal the letter up. Address it to yourself. Put a stamp on it. Give it to a trusted person in your life. Give them instructions on when to mail it to you.

Then, forget about it.

Don't worry, the next chapter will still be here when you finish.

You can do this now.

*I'll wait.*

# [ 21 ]

# WHY DID YOU STOP TRUSTING YOURSELF?

From one light topic to another. We're shifting from talking about death to talking about trauma. *But don't skip this chapter just because you think you haven't had any trauma.*

The kind of trauma I'm referring to is as inevitable as death. This chapter is for you if when you filled out the *Self-Trust Map + Scale*, you didn't rate your Self-Trust at a 10.

This book is filled with ways to help you rebuild trust in yourself, but why did you lose it in the first place?

This is not a practice of getting lost in the "Land of Conjecture" or wasting all day ruminating on *"Why? Why? Why?!"*

You don't have to spend years excavating all your past trauma. In fact, I encourage you NOT to do that. But often, when you have a general understanding of when, how, and why you lost trust in yourself, the path back to Self-Trust can be illuminated. And your path is going to be unique to you. Not everyone lost

Self-Trust the same way, so the return paths will also look different.

*Ask yourself:*

- When did I stop trusting myself?
- Why did I stop trusting myself?
- What happened that broke the trust in myself?
- Did I ever trust myself?

Spend some time reflecting in your journal. Or go on a hike with these questions. Notice what arises from within. What answers does your body and your soul already know?

I've asked this question a lot. Not surprisingly, the answers have varied. For some people, there was a specific moment in time when the trust in themselves was ruptured. A moment etched in time when a belief was implanted that they couldn't keep themselves safe. A belief that they made the "wrong decision" and couldn't trust what they thought they knew. An experience that registered as traumatic, that their body held onto for decades.

> **Maybe it was coming out of a toxic relationship and questioning yourself – *"How could I have let myself get into that situation?"***
>
> **Possibly creating a narrative that you can't trust your instincts about people moving forward so it's better to trust no one.**

For others, it was more gradual. A little messier and more confusing. The trust was chipped away at, slowly over time. Sometimes, without the person even realizing it. And it doesn't always have to be some big traumatic thing that happened when you lost trust in yourself.

> **More times than I can count, I've heard the story of a child walking into a room as their parents had just been fighting. Feeling the tension in their cells. The body signaling - *something* is wrong.**
>
> **But then, the well-intended parents contradict the body's messages and say, *"Everything is fine!"***

Do you believe what your gut is telling you?

Or do you believe the people who are required for you to stay alive? Pushing down and learning to disregard what your body is telling you.

*When you first stop trusting yourself, it's often out of survival.*

---

While there can be many reasons you lose trust in yourself, there is one I want to focus on in this chapter, because it comes up so frequently in my work. The 'T' word again. A buzzword that people have many definitions for.

**Trauma.**

- Trauma can disconnect you from your body.
- Trauma can disconnect you from your intuition.
- Trauma can have a huge impact on you if you can trust yourself.

But let's make sure we're on the same page when we're talking about what trauma is. Remember, don't skip this chapter just because you "haven't had any trauma".

The definition of trauma I'm referring to comes from Dr. Peter Levine, founder of *Somatic Experiencing*, and his research on animals in the wild. He explains that *anything* that overwhelms our nervous system's ability to cope *can be* registered as traumatic.

Anything that is too much, too soon, or too fast.

It's not about the specific event itself. It's about the impact on the nervous system and the support you receive afterwards. *Or, lack thereof.*

When your nervous system is overwhelmed, it goes into survival mode. This means the survival energy of the fight, flight, or freeze response, gets activated. And if the survival energy doesn't have a chance to move through and be discharged from your body, it can get "stuck" in your system.

**Unprocessed Trauma = Dysregulation in the Nervous System**

There will be an entire section later in the book exploring nervous system regulation. For now, I just want to focus on how unprocessed trauma can impact your Self-Trust.

There are often really good reasons someone disconnects from their physical body and their intuition. It often starts as protection. But once you've been disconnected for a while, it can feel scary to try to reconnect with your body. It starts to feel safer to make decisions solely from your logical brain or entirely based on external voices. Turning over your authority to an "expert" outside of you, instead of going inside to listen.

Understanding if trauma and disconnection from the body played a role in why you stopped trusting yourself is helpful because it links you to a pathway *back* to Self-Trust.

And it's a pathway I'm very familiar with.

I also want to be clear, I'm not defining any one specific experience as "trauma" for you. It's not my role to tell you if something was or wasn't traumatic for you.

Specifically right now, I'm speaking to experiences that led you to disconnect from your body. Because...

> If you experienced something that led you to disconnect from your body.
>
> It might've started to feel safer to stay disconnected.
>
> Therefore, a good place to start the return journey back to yourself is by *reconnecting* to the body.

But we can't speed through the reconnection process.

We have to move at the *"Speed of Trust"* which is often much slower than our logical brain wants to move. This is when titration comes in again.

Because even with the best intentions for reconnection, healing practices that don't consider a slow and curious pace can still be registered as "too much, too soon, or too fast" when not done intentionally.

Don't worry, you don't have to have it all figured out.

Just notice if disconnection from your body might be part of why you stopped trusting yourself. Acknowledge it. That's enough for one day.

[ 22 ]

# RAISED TO HUSTLE

June 1st

Could there be a shadow side to hard work?

I've literally never even considered this before. How is that possible?

I've had a few instances come up recently that have had me re-thinking my previously unexamined relationship with "hard work".

In many ways, I've learned to trust myself BECAUSE I've proven to myself I'll work hard at whatever it is I'm striving for. Sometimes, to a fault.

And I'm grateful hard work was instilled in

me from literally every possible caregiver in my life...

But again, could there actually be a shadow side to all of this?

I know that building any business takes a certain amount of hard work.

I trust myself to build a business with hard work as the only foundation. I've done it before. I could build this next business the same way.

But, do I trust myself to run this business differently?

Honestly? No...

Not yet.

I closed down my therapy practice because I want to do life differently now. And if I want a different life, I have to do business differently too.

My growth edge right now is not, "How can I work harder?"

My lesson right now is...

"Can I receive, even when it's easy?"

## [ 23 ]

# INTENTIONAL LIVING

Another way to talk about all the benefits of finding the golden skeleton key is to talk about having the confidence to live an intentional life. Living intentionally means knowing WHY you're making the decisions you're making.

**Simply put: It's life... On purpose.**

- *It's not a prescriptive life. It's the life YOU choose.*
- *It's the opposite of an unexamined life on autopilot.*

It takes bringing your thoughts, beliefs, and feelings into conscious awareness. And making decisions deliberately.

Lack of confidence can be a big barrier to living life this way. It takes a lot to stand up to the status quo and question the scripts you've been handed about how you should live.

Sometimes, it takes immense courage to live a life that YOU really want. A life that is aligned with what's right for you, regardless of what other people think.

At times, it can be tempting to follow the well paved path ahead of you. The path that's already illuminated from someone else's journey. And the promise of "belonging" that accompanies the path.

Even if that kind of belonging isn't *true* belonging.

It's brave to slow down and question if the life you're living is *actually* working for you. So, if you're in the early stages of this. KUDOS TO YOU!

I know it's hard. It does get easier (and then harder) and then really fucking great.

## [ 24 ]
## TO THE TRAILBLAZERS

There are downsides to living an intentional life though. It takes way more effort and energy to blaze your own trail. To question your past decisions and be deliberate about your choices moving forward.

*Especially* when you're first starting out.

Even though I've sat in tens of thousands of therapy sessions during my career, I can still poignantly remember some of them. Vivid moments forever etched in my soul. One, in particular, has been on repeat in my mind lately. Probably because what I said to her has been the same reminder I've repeatedly needed to hear over the past year.

She vulnerably shared her big and "audacious" dream with me. She let me in on her soul's calling. The "assignment" she couldn't get away from.

Her passion was palpable. Infectious even.

*Damn, I have such a cool job.*

This is truly where the magic is. The space in the Venn diagram, where the known meets the unknown. Where the seen intersects with the unseen. When we get to experience this overlap, it's visceral.

*Trailblazer, pay attention when you feel it.*

In our session, she relayed to me some of the feedback she'd gotten from other people her about her idea. And the common message from everyone?

They didn't get it.

And they definitely didn't understand why she'd even consider leaving something stable and predictable to follow this "thing" that didn't even make sense. And *their* inability to see *her* vision, was tempting her to pull the emergency brake.

She doubted herself. She questioned what she knew inside to be true. She bargained with herself to go back to the familiar path she'd been on before.

And, the parts of her that wanted her to return to the small box she'd lived her life in - made convincing points. They tried to seduce her with "logic" and "reason".

Even their facial expressions were in cahoots with her fears.

What I eventually said to her, is the same reminder I've told myself recently:

> "They're not supposed to 'get it' right now. It's not for them. It's *your* vision. If they 'got it' right now, it'd be because it's already been done before."

*Trailblazer, this advice doesn't take away from the fact that eventually it's really helpful to be able to describe your vision - for your vision to unfold.*

At some point, it will important to articulate concisely and confidently what your intuition is telling you.

But that doesn't mean the time is now.

It's okay, and likely necessary, to be in the messy stage of trusting for a while. You're the only one you have to convince to keep going.

*Trailblazer, you don't need other people to "get it" to trust yourself.*

## [ 25 ]

# HOW DO YOU KNOW THAT?

A barrier to living a life on purpose is not knowing *why* you're making the decisions you're making. How do you know what you know? Because someone told you? Or because you saw it with your own eyes? Here's a simple, yet often eye-opening practice to try. Make two lists:

| THINGS I KNOW BECAUSE I WAS TOLD | THINGS I KNOW BECAUSE IT'S WHAT I EXPERIENCED |
|---|---|

# [ 26 ]
# STUCK ON AUTOPILOT

"Is the life I'm living the same as the life that wants to live in me?"
- Parker Palmer

When we come into the world, we're handed a script for how to live life, as if we snagged the starring role in *Annie*. Or maybe *Hamilton*, or *Rent*. Or some other famous musical.

I call these *Life-Scripts*. And they can get in the way of living an intentional life. Primarily because, they don't often arrive on typed out paper to hold, examine, and make necessary edits to. There's no freedom to ad lib. We're expected to know our lines. And play our part.

> ***Life-Scripts*** **are the scripts we've been handed for our performance in life. Often without our conscious awareness, they instruct us on how we should live, love, work, and do life.**

They tell us what we should (and shouldn't) do.

Not everyone's scripts are the same though. We're assigned different parts to play depending on our family of origin and generation we're born into. And depending on the culture, schooling, religion, and political affiliation of those around us, we're assigned different musicals altogether.

**Are any of these *Life-Scripts* familiar to you?**

- Graduate high school and go directly to college.
- Get on the "Relationship Escalator" and don't get off until you find your husband.
- "Settle down" and live in one place.
- Start popping out babies right away.
- Follow the "gender roles".
- Get the job and work hard to build up a 401k so you can retire at 65.
- Subscribe to "hustle culture" and work really hard.
- Reject "hustle culture" and learn to rest.

**Or what about these messages, possibly handed down from family?**

- Make sure you can financially support yourself. Don't ever rely on a man.
- You should stay home with the kids - your husband should be the one to provide financially.
- Divorce is failure.
- Rich people don't care about other people.
- Don't make other people uncomfortable by talking about your feelings. Bottle everything up!
- Resting is lazy.
- It's weak to ask for help.

These *Life-Scripts* also want to tell you exactly how you "should" handle transitions in life. They instruct you how you're supposed to think, feel, and act when you're going through a divorce. After you have a baby. When someone you love dies. When you change jobs. Or receive a health diagnosis.

It's the instruction manual you didn't ask for.

These scripts can be sneaky too. Infiltrating your life without realizing it. Telling you what foods to eat to be a "good person". How you should feel about your body and sexuality. Constantly instructing you to defer to experts outside of yourself. Even when your body is screaming something different.

This is why you can't live an intentional life AND run on autopilot. You don't get both.

---

**Pausing for a moment, what are some Life-Scripts you were handed that immediately come to mind?**

- What messages did you get from school?
- What messages did you get from your family?
- What messages did you get from a political party?
- What messages did you get from media?
- What messages did you get from your culture?
- What messages did you get from the commercials in between cartoons you watched growing up?
- What messages did you get about what you "should" or "shouldn't" do?
- What messages did you get about where your worth came from?

**Now, when you look at the list of *Life-Scripts* you created, what do you notice?**

- Are there any scripts that surprise you?
- Are there any that you immediately want to reject?
- Are there any that you immediately want to hold onto tightly?

---

*Life-Scripts* can be very appealing. The biggest reason for their appeal that I've seen is, they offer a perceived sense of safety. They offer a promise that if you follow the prescribed paths, you'll be happy! And you don't have to think much about it. You can just cruise on autopilot to a life of ease and contentment.

They also allow you to outsource your decisions. And when you do that, you don't have to take accountability for your own choices. That can be pretty tempting when Self-Trust is lacking.

But then, one day, you wake up and are unsure how you got where you are.

- You've been on auto-pilot.
- You haven't been present.
- You've been a passenger in your own life.
- You've had to abandon parts of yourself along the way.

**Have you slowed down long enough to wonder if the scripts you're following are actually working?**

This doesn't mean that all the scripts you've been provided are wrong or bad. Some of these scripts might end up being perfect for you. The key factor here is intentionality. Taking time to actually get curious if the scripts are working for you.

After careful consideration, maybe your life will end up looking exactly like the original scripts you were given.

And then again, maybe it won't.

Either way though, intentionally choosing a path feels a whole lot different. You'll know *why* you chose it. And you'll be an active participant in your own life. This is what living an intentional life is all about.

**Do you have any fears of going "off-script"?**

If so, you're not alone. It's what I notice most when people slow down and acknowledge the *Life-Scripts* they've been living by.

Fear creeps in...

Fear tries to keep us safe by keeping things familiar.

*Fears I often hear are:*

- Fear of being misunderstood and rejected.
- Fear that life will be "harder".
- Fear that "I don't really know what I actually want".
- Fear that I can't trust myself to make the "right" decision.
- Fear that I'll have to admit my mistakes.

Are any of these fears familiar to you?

**Are you ready to get to know your fears?**

*(If yes, great - hold tight for the next chapter.)*

A common response when we realize something isn't working, is to swing in the complete opposite direction. *Anybody else have a rebellious teenager inside?*

Imagine a pendulum swinging back and forth.

Between the extremes. All or nothing. Black or white.

We're trying to find balance in our system. It's a normal and predictable response. *But, it's not working.*

**Reminder:**

- Unconsciously following the *Life-Scripts* you were handed isn't choice.
- However, unconsciously rebelling and doing the opposite of the *Life-Scripts* you were handed, also, isn't choice.

It all comes back to choosing with intention.

"Saying everything and saying nothing are not the only options."
- Africa Brooke

I've been examining my own *Life-Scripts* for a while now. Yet some had still managed to slip through, undetected. Specifically, the scripts about what it means to be a "good person" and what I should do to prove I "care", given to me by:

- The profession I'd been in for over a decade and a half
- Political parties

And it has me reflecting on the impact of these messages, specifically as a woman.

It's not all new. Some of this reflection and unraveling has been going on for a couple of years. Some has been present since I first opened my practice and didn't offer all my services for free. But some of the most insidious scripts have only recently started to reveal themselves more clearly. I've been looking at the messages I've received about how to be a "good feminist" or "good liberal". Oftentimes, there has been an actual script written out on exactly what you are supposed to say to signal to others that *"I'm a person who cares"* and *"I'm a good person."*

I've seen it infiltrate the mental health space. Sometimes, slowly and covertly. Sometimes, with a big neon sign.

As someone who spends a lot of time in the nuanced space of "both/and" and encourages clients to tour there often; these shifts didn't sit well. They actually felt counter to the very messages being delivered. This prescription was being handed out by self-proclaimed experts, with moral superiority, telling everyone that there is only one way to be a good person. Speaking for entire groups of people. And if you don't follow this exact script without question, you're "bad." Along with many other out-group names.

**I felt myself internally resulting to old disclaimers in my mind:**

- **Disclaimer:** Please don't be offended!!
- **Disclaimer:** Please don't misunderstand me!!
- **Disclaimer:** Please see the nuance!!
- **Disclaimer:** Please don't cancel me!!
- **Disclaimer:** Please still think I'm a "good person"!!

It was exhausting to try so hard *not* to be misunderstood. Convincing myself I owed "everyone" complete access to my nuanced inner dialogue anytime I shared something from my personal experience.

Maybe I could've stayed in the therapy space and challenged the unhelpful shifts I was noticing from within. I guess I could have. But honestly, I didn't want to.

Instead of playing by someone else's "house rules" or trying to get them to change the rules, I decided to just leave the house.

I've got my own house now. People who want to come visit me here, can. It's not the right house for everyone. And it doesn't need to be. That wouldn't even be practical. Plus, I'm a big fan of minimalism.

[ 27 ]

# INVITE YOUR FEARS TO TEA

In the last chapter, we talked about getting to know your fears as they arise. This is my absolute favorite practices to share with others and actually do, myself. Get ready to have tea with your fears... and see how much less scary they become.

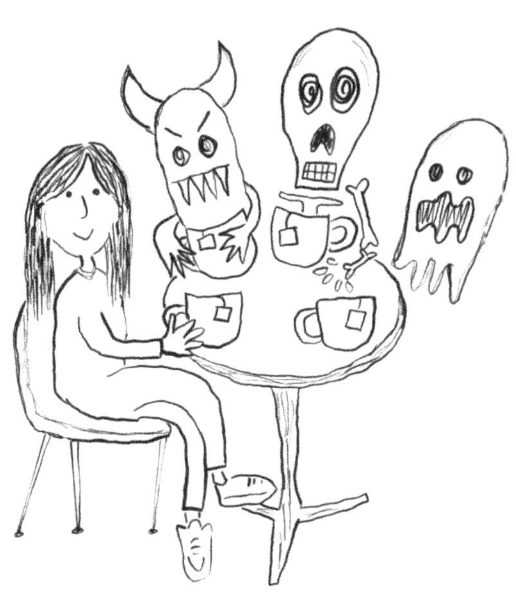

When you first notice fear arise, get curious about *how* the fear shows up. Is it:

- Physical sensations
- Mind chatter
- Distraction
- Doomsday future-tripping
- *Something else?*

Now, imagine what the fear looks like. Personify it. Allow the image of your fear to form in your mind's eye. Give it a name.

Next, invite the fear to be present with you, without trying to change it. Offer it some tea, like you would an old friend dropping by for a chat. *Seriously, brew two cups of tea. Sit down and drink the tea with your fear.*

Get to know how your fear takes her tea. *Two sugars and a splash of cream?*

Go slow, get curious. Ask the fear:

- "What are you trying to tell me?"
- "What do you want me to know?
- "What do you think would happen if you stopped being so afraid?"
- "What would happen if I didn't listen to you?"

Listen, without agenda.

Let your fear know you're not trying to get rid of it. You just want to understand it more so you can make the best decision.

Finally, express gratitude towards your fear. Thank if for joining you and offer a reminder... *you're welcome back anytime.*

[ 28 ]

# NATURE CLARITY

"A walk in nature walks the soul back home."

-Mary Davis

A simple, yet profound way to know if you're operating from a *Life-Script* is to get into nature. When you take a day or week or month to disconnect from the external world and connect to the rhythm of nature, clarity emerges as a byproduct. (*Sometimes after painstaking confusion, but still it often emerges.*)

You start to sense the difference between what you're doing because:

- You *actually* want to.
- You think it's what you *should* do.

If, after the past couple of chapters, you're struggling to know what *Life-Scripts* you're operating from, I encourage you to prioritize time alone in nature. As much as you can.

# [ 29 ]
# WHEN OUTSOURCING MAKES SENSE

Change and transformation are energetically draining. Whether it's the kind of change you choose, like getting pregnant, accepting a promotion, or moving across the country for your dream job.

Or, if you're experiencing something you'd never consciously choose that requires you to transform into the next evolution of yourself, like getting a cancer diagnosis, getting laid off, or becoming a caregiver to your dying spouse.

I wrote this entire chapter, to drill home an important message:

> **When you're exhausted and energetically drained from navigating life changes and messy seasons of evolution, it makes sense that you'd want someone else to take the lead and make decisions for you.**

I noticed this a lot in the chronic health space. Both in myself and with clients. The medical system is nothing short of exhausting. Whether it's the Western medical model prescribing the latest pill or an Eastern holistic approach searching for a root cause. And, maybe especially, when you're trying to combine the best of both healing worlds.

**It. Is. Exhausting.**

It makes so much sense that there will be periods when all you want to do is turn your decision making authority over to a person in a white coat. Or a shaman in the Peruvian jungle. Or a "shaman" in California.

**It makes sense. The impulse to outsource makes sense. *You* make sense.**

It's energy conservation.

And maybe, that's exactly what you need at different points along the way. To let someone else make some of your decisions. To alleviate the energetic burden of doing your own research on absolutely every single option. To allow yourself to receive. To know there are people that genuinely want to help and have your best interest at heart. To let go of the story that you have to do absolutely everything on your own.

That's why there's an entire chapter later on dedicated to the fundamental belief that *The Self-Trust Model* exists to not only empower you to trust *yourself* more, but to also help you learn to trust *others* (who have earned your trust). This framework takes into consideration that connection is our lifeline and we're not meant to do life (and all decision making) alone.

One more time...

**This shit is hard. You make sense.**

# [ 30 ]
# CONSCIOUS TRANSITIONS

"Transformation doesn't ask that you stop being you. It demands that you find a way back to the authenticity and strength that's already inside you. You only have to bloom."
-Cheryl Strayed

When you go through any transition in life, it's an opportunity for "old stuff" to get stirred up. Anything from your past that hasn't been tended to or processed, can bubble up to the surface. This is one reason big life transitions can cause so much stress. They can look (and feel) really messy.

During my therapy career, I often worked with people in these bardos. They were straddling two worlds. Between what used to be and what was still to come. Often, they were overwhelmed and disoriented at the intersection of life.

This is often when I'd hear from people who "didn't have trauma". They thought they were coming to therapy to deal with the stress of a new job, a move across the country, caring for an aging parent, a new baby, or a recent loss. All that was there. But what they discovered underneath, was so much more.

- Things they thought they were "over".
- Things that happened "so long ago".
- Things that "weren't a big deal".
- Things that had been buried deep inside.

Transitions can be powerful portals for reflection. They can be an opportunity to deliberately choose your path forward to become *more* of who you really are. When you approach a life transition with intention and conscious awareness, it can become a catalyst for more Self-Trust. Not just a stressful time you have to endure.

What I notice about these magical time warps is that words can sometimes fall short. But the *body*, is clear.

*What might it look like for you to bring conscious awareness to a current transition in life you're going through?*

---

**Here are two things I've learned about myself by navigating transitions in entrepreneurship:**

1. It's really hard to compartmentalize my "personal growth" from my "business growth" when so much of what I do for work is personal. Unfortunately, it's never about finding the one perfect marketing strategy to quickly turn the business into what I envision. The real work is tending to the deeper personal layers that always reveal themselves to be tangled up with my business.

- Beliefs around worth & career.
- Pattern of doing things alone and never asking for help.
- Difficulty receiving from others.
- Old stories about what happens if you slow down.
- Beliefs around motherhood & business.

2. I don't tend to stick to just one big lift transition at a time. I like to pile up the bardos - one on top of another.

At thirty-seven, I've spent most of my adult life undecided about whether to become a mom or not. I ended a good marriage to my best friend because of this indecision . But for the past couple of years - my indecision has been shifting... towards desire.

I've also consciously entered into a new partnership (*sometimes painstakingly conscious*). This partnership has come with a new role for me. Not just as a wife. But also, as a bonus mom. Or as they call me, *Maddy*.

It's the first time I've had to consider other people when it comes to my business. I don't get to lone-wolf it anymore. Part of me welcomes this. Another part doesn't know how to let go of my solitary and fiercely independent tendencies. She's holding a death grip on how I used to be successful in business. Here's what I know:

- This is the work I know I want to avoid.
- This is the work I know is mine to do.
- This is the work I know is required to get what I claim to want.

# [ PART 2 ]
# SUMMER

We continue... with the essence of the **Summer Solstice.**

A celebration of nature.

A revisiting of the intentions set in Spring.

A commitment to the hard work required with longer days.

A spontaneous exhale as your body expands into the rays of the sun's medicine.

A time to water the seeds.

A time to salute the sun.

A magical day of light.

Digging into the depths of the concepts and "doing the work"...

The meat of the book...

Illuminating what you most need to see and tend to...

. . .

And we persevere through the long days.

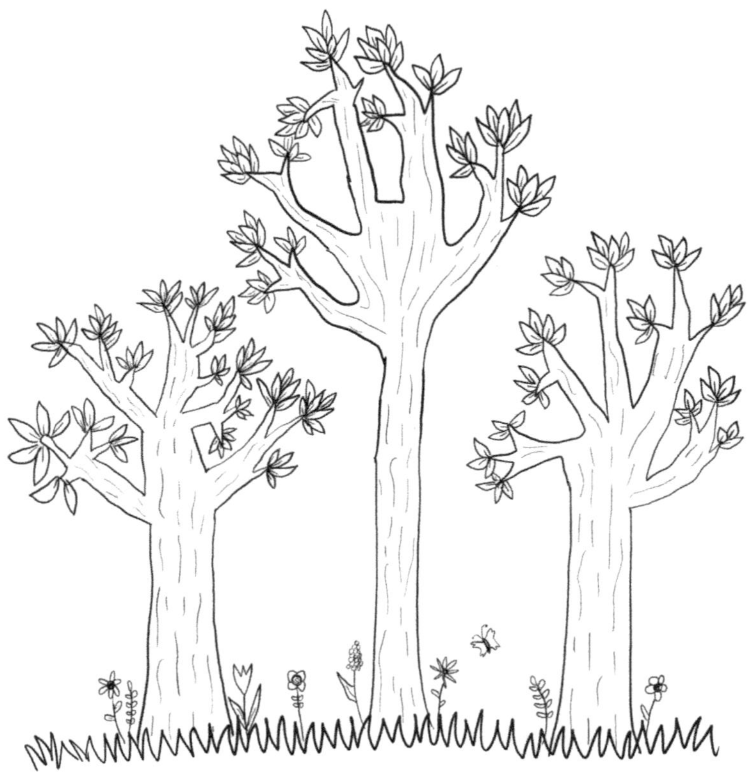

[ 31 ]

# THIS ISN'T IT

June 20th

Okay, I'm going to finally write the thing I've been feeling since the second session of the online group I've been running – but didn't want to be true.

It doesn't feel like I expected it to. And not in a "Oh how wonderful, this is surpassing my expectations kind of way!"

This group... is NOT it.

The women are great. The content is great.

But it doesn't light me up the way Adventure Club or individual therapy did.

I really wanted this group to be the answer.

But wanting something to be true... doesn't make it so.

Today, as I was prepping for a fire ceremony inside the group... I got to thinking about my mushroom experience from last month.

The message that came through about my business had been intense, but I'd tried to brush it off: "BURN IT ALL DOWN!"

I had assumed Mama Shroom was being a bit hyperbolic. I'm sure I wasn't supposed to <u>actually</u> burn down everything in my business and start fresh. I'm sure she didn't <u>actually</u> mean I needed to cancel all upcoming groups for the year and start my email list at zero. That'd be crazy.

Mama Shroom speaks in metaphor - I was certain that's all it was...

Now... I'm not so sure.

I still don't know what's going to happen with "The 13 Lessons". But today, I'm admitting to myself that this online group isn't going to be the path for my new business.

Here's to continuing to show up, even when it doesn't makes any sense. And trusting that it will... eventually.

[ 32 ]

# LEARNING TO RECEIVE

"We don't reach the mountaintop from the mountaintop. We start at the bottom and climb up. Blood is involved."
- Cheryl Strayed

Earlier, I shared how I'm grateful for the work ethic instilled in me. It's what I've credited any success I've ever had in life to. Any accomplishment I reached, I attributed it to how hard I worked to achieve it.

I've long glorified hard work. And revered the *people* who work hard.

I grew up on an ever-expanding crop farm outside of a small town in Kansas. Primarily raised by my farmer dad, I don't have the same childhood memories of summer that many of my friends do. I didn't associate summer with long pool days, excitement to be out of school, and walks to the snow cone shop with friends.

Until I had my own pick-up and could escape for a different kind of hard work with basketball practice and weekend tournaments; summer meant longer days for all the work farm life requires.

Driving the grain cart for wheat harvest, farm chores, taking care of the animals, and mowing. Always...

So. Much. Mowing.

There was so much to mow that even when we did it every day, by the time we "finished" it was time to start over again.

Farming runs on both sides of my family as far back as I'm aware of. Now, while I can't remember a single conversation when any of my parents or grandparents talked about our family values, I know without a doubt the one value was universally passed down out of necessity...

Hard work.

It was a value so baked into the culture of farming and my family, my ancestors probably assumed it was just an integral character trait they couldn't get rid of - even if they wanted to.

Or at least, that's how *I* felt about it. Because let's be real, my ancestors were so busy just surviving off the land - they didn't have time to sit around self-reflecting or philosophizing about life. That's a privilege they provided for me through their generations of hard work.

**(Thank you, thank you, thank you - by the way...)**

I'd spent my entire life assuming that having a strong work ethic was purely and unequivocally "good." It was maybe the only thing I could consistently rely on that made me a "good person." My value and my worth - fully tied up with how hard I worked.

**But what if... that shadow side I alluded to earlier was also real?**

What if, just like everything else in the world, there's another perspective to consider...

If that *were* true, it wasn't a perspective I was necessarily interested in exploring. My identity was *so* wrapped up in being a hard worker. Perceiving success as intrinsically tied to my work ethic. What would happen if I start to unravel that?

No thanks.

This is why I have so much compassion for those who don't want to explore the scripts they were handed in life. I understand why it can feel threatening to their very existence. And it's tempting to follow the path laid out ahead of them.

---

The moment I decided to be disciplined in my business and focus only on "The 13 Lessons" - the unraveling began.

> **What if I'd been using hard work as a shield my entire life?**

A few months into this uncomfortable process, I listened to a podcast episode about hard working and high achieving, career women. And an uncomfortable seed was planted.

*Lacey Sites*, on her podcast *LITerally*, began talking about how in her business-coaching business, she sees high achieving women use hard work or over-working as an "apology to the world." She went on to describe how women often "justify" their success by proving how hard they worked to achieve it.

God forbid you might actually be talented at something. Or have a natural inclination. Or your enjoyment for something actually makes you better at it. **If your success makes someone else uncomfortable, you can soothe them (and yourself) by explaining just how hard you worked for it.**

She went on to ask a question into the void of the podcast listeners - an arrow directly at my shield of hard work.

*What if hard work isn't the secret to your success?*

What?!

What would that even mean? Of course hard work is the reason I've been successful.

Her language about having a "natural inclination" sparked a particular memory in me. I vividly remember the weekend I began my *Somatic Experiencing* (*SE*) training. It was the first snowy day in February. In a barn outside Bozeman, Montana where people would go cross country skiing on lunch breaks.

I remember the resonance I felt in my body as I learned about the basics of this trauma resolution modality – *which I'll explain in more detail later in this book.* By this point in my career, I'd been trained in many models of therapy. Some resonated, some didn't. But nothing had felt quite like this before. Everything I was learning about and then practicing in the break out groups felt like a "coming home". There was a framework and a language that captured how I intuitively worked with clients. Things made sense in a new way.

As I was writing about *SE* for this book, I revisited my oversized binder full of years of training, practice, and notes from my internal process. I found a note I'd written after receiving feedback from the trainer. After our first practice session, she'd wanted to share praise and her perspective that I was a "natural fit" with *SE*.

I worked hard to take in the compliment. Because from my perspective, I actually agreed. But giving myself credit didn't come easy. I couldn't deny it though. I witnessed other people struggle in the practice sessions. But I didn't feel their same pain points. Working this way actually *did* feel natural and there was a sense of ease to it.

The *LITerally* podcast episode had me questioning...

> *What was so bad about going towards the thing I'm good at?*
>
> *Did I always have to choose the harder path?*

I think I was a good somatic therapist because I prioritized learning from mentors who I respected, I put in a great deal of time and effort, I practiced, and, yes, I worked hard. All of this is true.

And.

I also had a natural tendency to want to work with people in that way. And it allowed for my starting point to be different from some other people.

**OH MY GOD, even as I type this now – my whole body cringes.**

I'm fine telling you about how hard I worked to be a good somatic therapist. But not that I have any natural ability for it.

I think Lacey was onto something...

Here are some other questions to ponder if any of this chapter resonates with you:

- How are you trying to make your success more comfortable for others?
- What would happen if you let yourself have a natural ability towards something?
- What would happen if you let something be "easy"?
- What if your success is actually in *spite* of your over-working patterns?
- Who are you afraid will be triggered by your success?
- Do you feel deserving of success that comes "easy" to you?
- Can you lean into the parts of your life that come with ease?

# [ 33 ]
# THE SELF-TRUST COMPASS

I know how disorienting, messy, confusing and downright terrifying the transitions we go through in life can be. They can turn our world upside down. They can crack us open in the most unimaginable ways. Especially when they are the *before/after* kind of change.

Transitions can rock us to our very core and send us on the trajectory of rock bottom. I have no way of preventing you from reaching that cave of dark despair. *I'm not even sure I would if I could.*

Sometimes... it's the only option.

But my hope is... if you happen to find yourself on a dark-night-of-the-soul journey, you can reach for the compass I gave you earlier.

And have a way to orient back to yourself, even in the darkness.

Back to the voice inside, even when she's just a whisper.

Because even though there's not a bypass route to a life full of purpose and confidence, you also don't have to glamorize the "struggle path" for the sake of the "struggle story". You can choose to learn from those who have traversed these trails before you and allow the compass to support your journey.

*The Self-Trust Compass* is here to make things simpler, while never claiming it will be easy. It's here to provide helpful structure to guide and orient you while leaving plenty of space for curiosity, flexibility, and the freedom to choose your own path.

**Here it is again...**

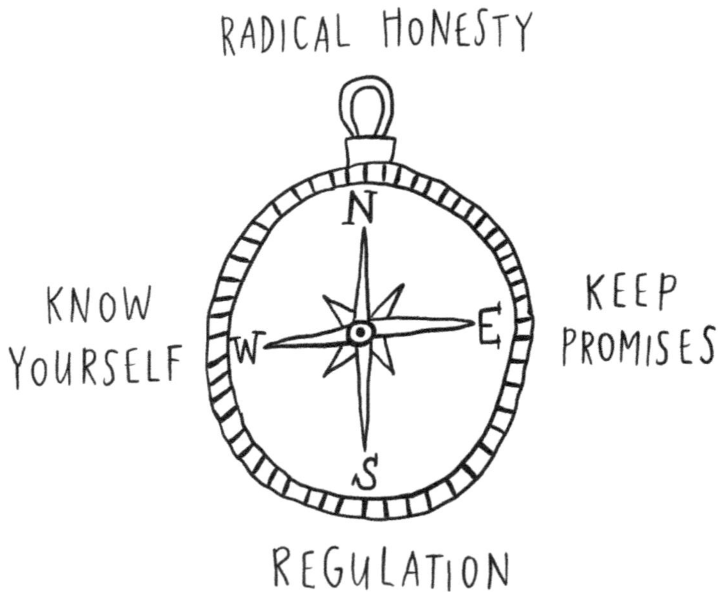


This is the framework for building more Self-Trust so that you can confidently choose the life you want to live. With all the directions of *The Self-Trust Compass*, it's helpful to do this work in layers. The directions are not a checklist where things get marked off once and are done forever. You'll move around the compass continually. Each time you revisit a direction, you'll be able to go a deeper layer in.

**North - Radical Honesty:**

(*Likely a good place to start if you're lost or just starting out*)

Trustworthy people tell the truth. If you want to trust yourself, you can't lie to yourself. This direction is all about going inward and getting real with yourself. Being truly honest about where you are, how you got there, and where you want to go.

**East - Keep Promises**:

Trustworthy people do what they say they are going to do. Consistently, over time. When you habitually follow through on your commitments, you have no choice but to trust yourself. You do want to make sure you're keeping the "right" promises - *don't worry I'll tell you what I mean by that soon.*

**South - Regulation**:

Nervous System Regulation, that is. It's really difficult to trust your intuition when your nervous system is dysregulated. Start with the basics to access a baseline of regulation in your system: fuel (food + water), movement, sleep, sunlight, and connection (others + nature).

**West - Know Yourself:**

Self-awareness is a prerequisite to Self-Trust. You've got to stop being a stranger to yourself if you want to trust yourself. Slow down and get curious about yourself. Discover what might be underneath your initial reactions.

# [ 34 ]
# NORTH: RADICAL HONESTY

**How do you learn you can trust someone?**

They tell the truth. Even when it's uncomfortable.

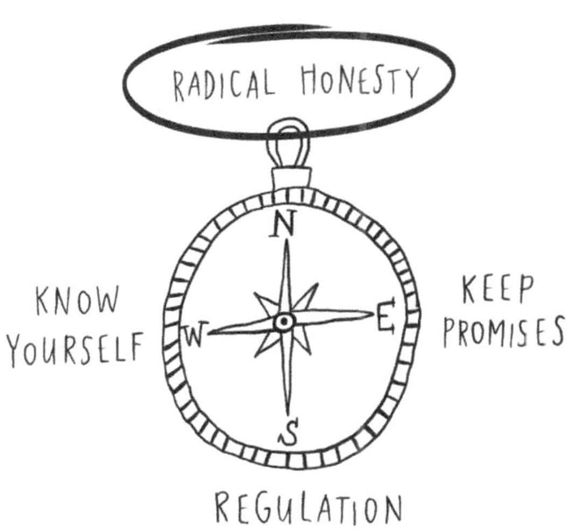

Yeah, I guess that sounds kinda obvious, right? We don't trust people who lie to us. Even when they have really good intentions for "skirting" around the truth. We learn we can trust someone when they are consistently honest with us. Especially when the truth might be uncomfortable to hear. *This is not an invitation to be an asshole. It is possible to be honest AND deliver it with kindness.*

The same applies to building trust with yourself. If you want to trust yourself more, you have to tell yourself the truth. Even when it's hard. Even when it's uncomfortable. Maybe even, *especially* when it's hard and uncomfortable.

**Here are 4 Signs it might be time to find North on your compass (and be Radically Honest with Yourself):**

1. You're just starting out on the Self-Trust journey.
2. You're lost, stuck, or confused about where you're headed in life.
3. You're "spinning your wheels" and "doing all the things" but not seeing the progress you want.
4. It's been a while since you intentionally found North.

*In this chapter, we'll start with the first two signs.*

### 1. You're just starting out on the Self-Trust journey.

Before you begin any adventure, it can be really helpful to identify your starting point. Whether it's a metaphorical journey to trusting yourself more or a very practical journey to a different part of the world. You need to first find the 'You Are Here' pin on the map. We did this with the *Self-Trust Map + Scale* in chapter 18.

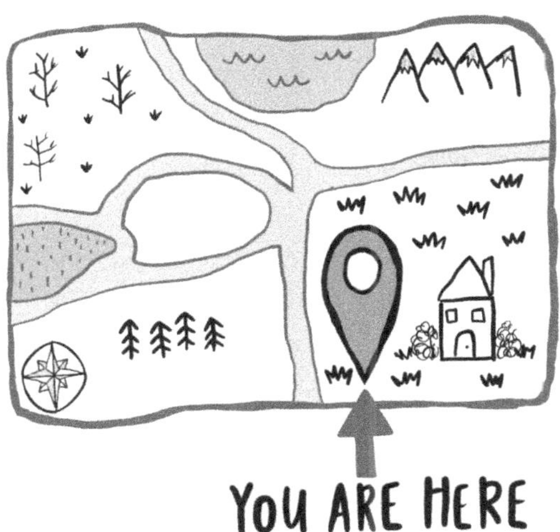


If you're trying to get to Kansas City, you need to know if you're starting out in Southern California or beginning your journey from Chicago. The adventure will look different depending on your starting point. And the resources you'll need will be different. **Being honest with yourself at the beginning is a way to set yourself up for success.**

On the journey to trusting yourself more, lining up the compass arrow to point North looks like getting radically honest about your current level of Self-Trust. Because if you're longing for something different in life, it's helpful to first identify what it is you're already doing.

We've already explored a lot of these ideas, but here's a reminder of ways to begin your Self-Trust journey:

- What is your current level of Self-Trust? See *Self-Trust Map + Scale.*
- When/How/Why did you stop trusting yourself?

- Has anything new been illuminated for you?
- In what ways are you outsourcing your life?
- Where are you listening to someone else tell you what to buy, what to watch, what to put into your body, etc
- What *Life-Scripts* are you unconsciously following?
- What "internalized should's" are influencing your decisions?
- Where are you turning over your power to someone else?
- Who are the "experts" you're trusting in life?

It's possible to lose trust in yourself in "big" moments. There are many "Crisis of Trust" moments that we can all experience:

- Betrayal
- Health Scare
- A traumatic loss
- Becoming a parent
- Questioning a part of your identity

But often, it's the "little" moments that can gradually chip away at the trust you have in yourself. Piece by piece. Without even realizing it. Every moment you override what your body is trying to tell you. Every time you disconnect from your emotions and your intuition; you disconnect from yourself a little bit more too. You drown out the inner voice of wisdom. What started as protection, can become a cage.

People have different wounds around Self-Trust. Therefore, the return journeys are also going to be unique. This is why identifying your starting point is critical. Otherwise, you're following someone else's path and hoping for the best.

"If you can see the path laid out in front of you step-by-step, it's probably someone else's."
- Joseph Campbell

**2. You're lost, stuck, or confused about where you're headed in life.**

The land of *Radical Honesty* is a great place to visit when you know something in your life is out of alignment. *Something* isn't working. You're lost. Finding North on a compass when you're lost can be grounding and can offer the much-needed hope of survival. Once you line up the compass needle and know which direction you're facing, you've got a chance of survival. You can exhale.

Self-Trust isn't an "all or nothing" thing.

You might have some areas in your life where you are connected to yourself and trusting your decisions. While in another area, you're constantly second-guessing and doubting yourself. I see this all the time. *I've worked with a ton of women who are crushing it in their careers, and struggling in their romantic relationships*.

Part of the process of being radically honest is looking at the different aspects of your life and identifying where you have trust in yourself and where you don't. This assessment of where you have more Self-Trust and less Self-Trust, helps guide your individual journey. Look at these areas of your life, and get real with yourself:

- Relationships
- Career
- Health

- Finances
- Living Situation

This includes looking at your internal circumstances in each area *and* the external. You may *want* to not have a health issue or physical limitations. You might *want* to be in a different body that doesn't experience pain. You might *want* the person you love to still be alive. You might *want* to not live in systems that are oppressive.

But merely *wanting* something doesn't make it the reality.

If you don't acknowledge the reality of your external and past experiences, your path forward is skewed. You don't live in a vacuum.

I'd make a case that there's a time and place to be a little delusional when you're chasing big dreams in life. But this isn't it. It's important to be honest about the systems and structures you currently exist in, so you can make the right changes.

Acknowledging the reality of your circumstances is not meant to discourage you. It's actually the opposite. Understanding the reality of what's happening internally and externally can be an empowering process. Because then, you know the next steps available to you. **You're taking action, grounded in reality.**

[ 35 ]

# APPLYING RADICAL HONESTY

July 6th

I understand how sometimes the advice to live "as if" you already have the life you want to create, can be helpful.

It's that visualization, manifestation, and "woo" space that I'm sometimes into.

But NOW doesn't seem like the time for it.

I don't think over-extending myself financially to make myself "open" to the life I want - is the answer.

There's a time and place for everything. And NOW – seems like the time for radical honesty.

NOW seems like the time to be honest about the current realities of my business - not what I WANT to be the reality.

Here's one reality... I'm not making the same kind of money I was in my private practice. If I spend money as if I was, the savings I was able to accumulate during that time, won't last very long.

Now is the time to be practical. To cut back on spending. To prioritize only what is necessary.

This honesty with myself - will give me the gift of time...

Time to write...

Time to see what all of this is meant to become...

Radical Honesty with myself gives me the gift of possibility.

The spacious gift to dream big and take chances.

To live the life that my soul wants to live.

Also... I'm not going to pretend making more money didn't make life easier. I liked making more money. It was a far cry from the penny pinching and working multiple jobs I've done my whole life. And the nervous system work I was doing around money was working. I was creating more space for money to come in.

I DO want to return to that. I miss gifting spa days to friends and not batting an eye at $8 matcha lattes.

One more thing, if I'm being really honest, that I've never had before, and is worth WAY more than financial security.

I have a husband who is delusionally supportive. Or at least, it used to seem delusional. From the moment I met him, he never thought my dreams were too big. He's never made me feel silly for wanting to do big things. In fact, when I first told him I wrote a very raw and shitty first draft of what could be considered a book. He didn't laugh. He didn't say what my mind was telling me - "Who the fuck are you to write a book?!".

Instead, he told me about the cover he imagined. The "best selling author" listed at the top. The book signings. The people that would be impacted.

He believed in my big ideas long before I did. Getting him on board with my dreams isn't a hurdle I have to clear. Halle-fucking-lujah!

[ 36 ]

# CHOOSE YOUR HARD

The third sign it could be helpful to return to North and be radically honesty with yourself is:

**3. You're "spinning your wheels" and "doing all the things" but not seeing the progress you want.**

If you find yourself here, you're probably exhausted. Because it "feels" like you're doing all the things you're "supposed" to do. You're taking action. You're doing things. *So why aren't you feeling better?*

Before we get into the possible 'why' underneath this, I want to first invite you to get radically honest. With facts.

- Start by gathering tangible data. What time, energy, and resources are you *actually* putting towards your goals?
- If you say you want to find a new job because your current one is causing too much stress in your life, how much time are you spending filling out applications and interviewing?

- What is your calendar telling you about your priorities?
- Objectively look at the progress you've made towards your goals. What movement have you made in the direction of your goals?
- Remember that healing isn't linear. There will be normal setbacks and hurdles. Do you need to give yourself more credit?
- You may need to find a new way of tracking progress around abstract goals like "more confidence", "less anxious", or being connected to your body.

**If, after all that radically honest reflection, you discover that you're *actually* putting in the time and effort required for change *and* you're truly not seeing progress, you might be misattributing the anxiety.**

Maybe you've been attributing your stress and anxiety and dissatisfaction in life to the job you've had for the past five years. The long hours and boss who doesn't see your potential. Then, you do all the work to finally leave. You get a new job. A new boss. You even get to work from home now. No commute and pajama pants all day.

*So why is that background hum of angst still there?*

*Why do you still have a pit in your stomach?*

Maybe, it wasn't entirely about your career. Maybe that was just the easiest place to attribute the stress. It was the obvious and convenient culprit of your anxiety. And it's not until you leave your job, dig into an even deeper layer of honesty with yourself, that you discover, it's actually been your *marriage* that wasn't working.

Working from home didn't solve that.

---

**Being radically honest with yourself is often hard.**

Sometimes it requires you to do a thing you really don't *want* to do:

- Set a boundary with a parent
- End a long term friendship
- Have a hard conversation that could fundamentally change your marriage
- Admit to yourself that you *don't* want to be a mom

These things are not easy for most people I know. In fact, I have a ton of compassion and understanding for people that never want to do personal growth work or go to therapy. Or be *this* honest with themselves. These people make a lot of sense to me. It can feel hopeless to acknowledge what might have to change in your life or admit where you've made a mistake.

But, I also know that *not* being radically honest with yourself - is also hard. A different kind of hard. And it just happens to be the kind of hard I'm no longer able to live with.

Not being honest with yourself is a kind of hard that eats away at your soul from the inside. The out-of-integrity kind of hard that feels like a life sentence of suffering.

Once you know, you can't *un*-know.

And finally, the fourth sign that it's time to orient towards North.

**4. It's been a while since you intentionally found North.**

Ongoing self-auditing is critical. Being honest with yourself is not something you do once and then check it off your to-do list forever. It's helpful to check in every once in a while and make sure you're still headed in the direction you want to go. To confirm the destination you chose at the beginning is still where you want to end up.

Checking in with yourself periodically allows you to pivot when you need to. Course correct before you're too far down a path. Once you start to connect to the voice of your inner wisdom, you can listen when she whispers. Instead of waiting until she screams.

Remember, this is hard work. Especially when you first start out. You might not have access to all the layers of truth in the beginning. Just start being honest. About small things. Mundane things. Silly things. Build up the habit of telling yourself the truth about if you want pizza or sushi for dinner.

Stop saying you're "fine", when you're not.

Sometimes you have to acknowledge an outer layer of truth, and take action. Before you can access the next layer. You can apply the concept of titration here. Little bits of honesty at a time. Giving yourself permission to work with just the first layer. And when you prove to yourself you can handle what comes with honesty, you can trust yourself to be honest about the next thing.

An outer layer to begin with is asking yourself:

***What fears do I have about being honest with myself?***

Maybe you're similar to some of the people I've worked with who answered:

- "I don't want to admit I've been living by what someone else says is best."
- "I know I'll have to do something different... and I'm not ready."
- "I'm going to lose my relationship with Billy."
- "I don't want to admit I messed up."

It comes back to **choosing your hard**. Because being radically honest is hard.

But choosing, even unconsciously, to live out of alignment with your integrity, is another kind of hard.

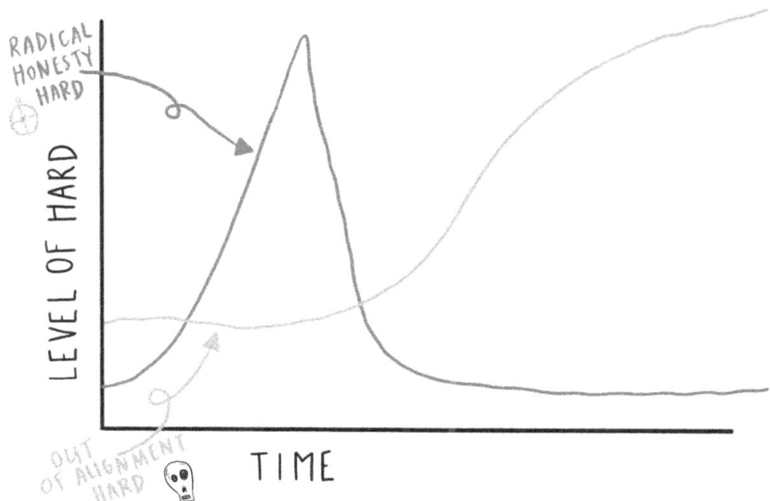

## [ 37 ]

# JUST FAKE IT

If "fake-it-till-you-make-it" strategies have actually worked for you long term to build genuine confidence, there's a good chance you're not reading this book.

But, if using "positive affirmations" and "fake it" strategies *did* help you to build lasting self-esteem and confidence - *and* you also made it this far into this book - feel free to skip this chapter. Enjoy your

*Here's my experience with this particular advice...*

Looking in a mirror and repeating words to myself I didn't believe never struck me as a solid game plan that would have lasting results. But I still gave it a shot - *many times.* For so long, I desperately wanted to feel confident. So, I tried all of the hacks and advice given by "confidence experts".

- Positive affirmations in the mirror? - ✔
- Power Pose? - ✔
- Pretending to feel confident? - ✔

- Making a list of my accomplishments and trying to "logic" my way to confidence? - ✔

I'm including this in the section of *Radical Honesty* because through this lens, it now makes sense to me why the "fake it" approach never worked for me. Or for so many other women who've also tried it. We created a narrative that something was wrong with *us* - instead of something being wrong with the approach.

At best, I've seen the "fake-it-till-you-make-it" approach have short lived results. It might be able to get you over the hump of a presentation or through a first date. But the results were never genuine confidence - radiating from within. There was always a level of incongruency.

If we're being radically honest, "faking it" is another form of lying. And even when you have the best intentions, you're still lying to yourself. And lying to yourself erodes trust in yourself. And lacking trust in yourself prevents true confidence from developing.

I've found there's a lot of truth in the old adage: *Honesty is the best policy.*

Even if the truth in the moment is:

- *"Part of me still doesn't believe I'm good enough."*
- *"I'm struggling right now to love myself."*
- *"My income isn't growing exponentially and I don't feel like a magnet for wealth."*

A fundamental aspect of *EMDR®* (*Eye Movement Desensitization and Reprocessing*) is that we have a deeply embedded negative belief that usually sounds something like:

- *"I'm not good enough."*
- *"I'm not worthy."*
- *"I'm too much."*
- *"I'm bad."*
- *"I'm not lovable."*
- *"I'm a failure."*

Once my clients were able to identify their core negative belief (*usually the one that made them want to throw up*), the most common thing I heard them say was:

> Pointing to their head: *"I **know** it's not true..."*
>
> Pointing to some other part of their body: *"...but it **feels** so true"*.

This is the incongruence I was referring to earlier. The gap between what your core wound *wants* you to believe and what you *know* to be true - is just too big to cross.

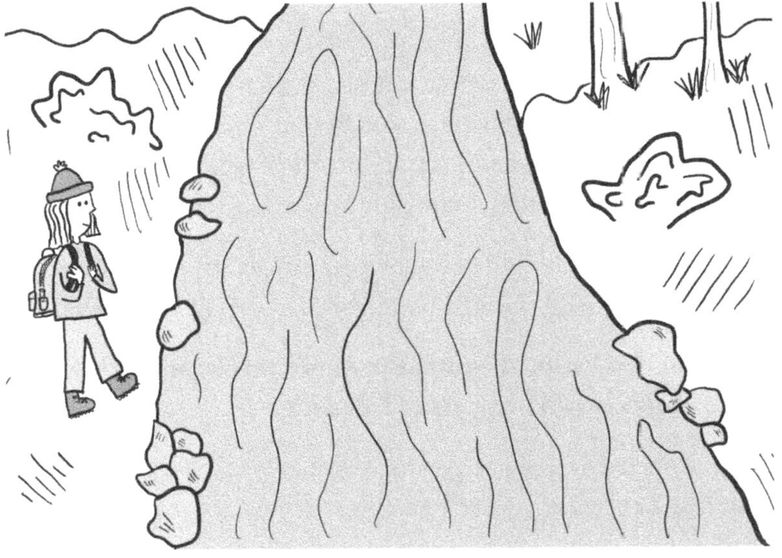

Even if you want to believe one of the counter positive beliefs:

- *"I'm good enough."*
- *"I'm worthy."*
- *"I'm lovable."*
- *"I know I can figure it out."*

When the negative belief is "stuck" in your physical body, it's hard to get your brain to budge on it.

*EMDR* has a specific protocol to follow in supporting a person to decrease the intensity of a negative belief - until it actually no longer *feels* true. And then, another process to "install" the more desirable positive belief.

Unfortunately, it was never as easy as just repeating the positive belief enough times.

There are other ways this negative-to-positive belief process can play out... genuinely. We'll explore many of them together in this book. But the key piece that all these processes have in common is they move at the *"Speed of Trust"*.

***"Speed of Trust"*** is not merely a cognitive experience of believing something. But it's actually an *embodied* experience of trust. Trust that some part of you *truly* believes what you're saying about yourself and your life - on a deep cellular level.

It doesn't mean that all parts of you are ready to immediately jump on board with the affirmation of: *"I'm a magnet for money!"*

**I know for me, I could never trick myself into believing something that I didn't.**

But through this work, a part of you begins to *actually* believe that you can trust yourself to have money (or whatever your goal affirmation is). I went through many stages of this when I was working to increase my capacity to hold wealth. Specifically, when it came to my finances as I began to grow my private practice. But I knew the concept of "wealth" wasn't limited to money.

Up until that time in my life, I'd always made a low salary, but I knew how to stretch a dollar. I had an extreme aversion to any "extras" I could avoid (like ATM fees), and actually *made* money by using my credit cards. I also had beliefs tied up in the narrative that making such a low wage actually made me a "better person".

Through this exploration, a mantra eventually arose into my consciousness from within myself. And I began to say it out loud to myself every day.

> **"Thank you for the financial prosperity and abundance. I know I can trust myself with wealth and I choose to live generously."**

It didn't matter if I'd just received a large deposit into my bank account. Or if it was during a rough drought of income.

This mantra was helpful to me - *because it came from me.*

It captured my genuine gratitude for what I already had, trust in myself to hold wealth of all kinds, and my desire to live with a generous heart. I began to actually chip away at the old narrative that having money made me selfish, entitled, or a bad person.

This is why I actually *do* encourage people to explore mantras. Because they are different from following a prescribed positive affirmation.

**Tips for Using Mantras:**

- Focus on mantras that genuinely arrive from within yourself. This doesn't mean you can't get ideas from other people – *I'm actually going to be prompting you with ideas for each of the 4 directions on The Self-Trust Compass*. But notice which mantras actually resonate as true already - in *your* body.
- Ensure at least *one* part of you believes the mantra. You might have other conflicting parts inside, who like to bring up all the reasons it's *not* true, that's okay. Just make sure some part of you actually buys into what you're saying to yourself. You might need to play around with the language until you get it right.
- Get curious about the parts of you who *don't* believe the mantra. These parts have crucial roles in your journey. They will shine the light on the true work that needs to be done in order to have the positive beliefs about yourself that you desire.
- Repetition. Find a time that makes sense for you to repeat the mantra to yourself every day. If you can, combine the mantra with another habit you do daily to increase the chance you actually remember to do it. *I repeated my money mantra each day as I looked at my bank account.*
- Breathe and notice your body as you repeat the mantra. Allow the mantra to expand to also include images, colors, emotions, and physical sensations. Allow yourself to have an embodied experience of the mantra. To truly *feel* it. Not just say it. While also tenderly holding the parts that don't fully trust yet. It's normal if the "*Speed of Trust*" takes longer than your logical brain wants it to.

At the end of each direction on *The Self-Trust Compass*, I'll provide a jumping off point for mantras. A few ideas to consider when you feel drawn to deepen your work in that direction.

[ 38 ]

# MANTRAS FOR RADICAL HONESTY:

- I will identify my starting point.
- I will be honest with myself. Even when it's uncomfortable. Especially when it's uncomfortable.
- I can only heal what I first acknowledge.

[ 39 ]

# COSMIC TREE RINGS

"The most courageous things I've ever done began with simply telling the truth, even when the truth meant something would end."
– Alix Klingenberg

Here is a practice to give you some structure in being radically honest with yourself.

This is more than just a cognitive exercise. To get the most out of it:

- Set aside an hour of undisturbed time.
- Put on some background music.
- Gather paper and markers.
- Brew yourself a cup of tea.
- Take a few breaths to land more fully in your body.
- And then... begin.

Choose an area of life you'd like to focus on. If you filled out the *Self-Trust Map + Scale*, you may want to focus on the specific area of your life you chose then. Or you can look at your life more holistically.

This is a practice you can come back to many times. The idea that you can never step into the same river twice. You will be a different person the next time you do this.

## COSMIC TREE RINGS

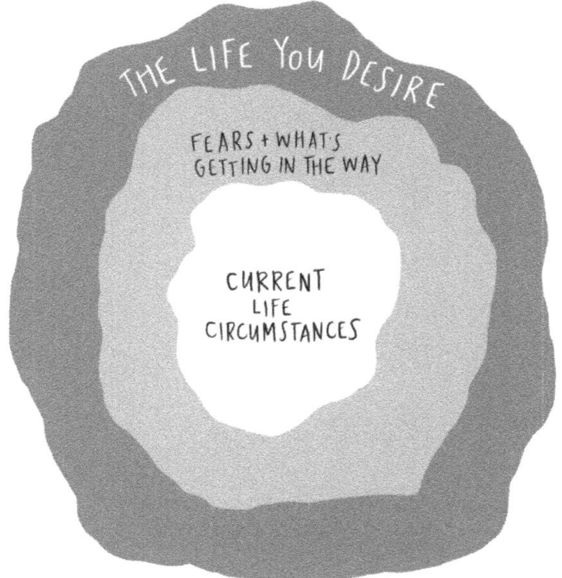


Starting with the inner ring of the circles. This is your starting point. Take a Radically Honest look at what your life looks like RIGHT NOW.

- What's working in your life? What's not?
- What's your current physical/emotional/relationship/financial state?
- What season of life are you in right now?
- How are you already living in alignment with your values + purpose? How are you not?
- Where do you trust yourself? Where don't you?

**Take your time. There's no rush.**

Then, explore the outer ring. This is the destination you aspire to reach. Be radically honest about what you *actually* want your life to be like. Hopefully, you've had some time leading up to this exercise to begin discerning between what *you* want and what you've been told you're supposed to want.

- What would your most expansive life look like?
- What hopes, dreams, and desires do you have for yourself and loved ones?
- What would it look like to be an active participant in your life?
- How would you be living if you really trusted yourself?
- Define what "more" in your life means to you.

**Pause. Take a breath. Take a stretch.**

And then, onto the middle ring. These are the fears that might be getting in your way from where you are to where you want to be.

- What changes would you have to make?
- What's getting in your way?

- What (or who) might you lose if you expand into the outer ring?
- What parts of yourself might not be able to go with you to the outer ring?
- Are you ready to grieve those parts that aren't coming?

There will always be a "path not taken". A "parallel life" you don't get to live because of the choices you made. Even when you make conscious decisions to go down a path you want, you may still want to make space to grieve the path you'll no longer get to live.

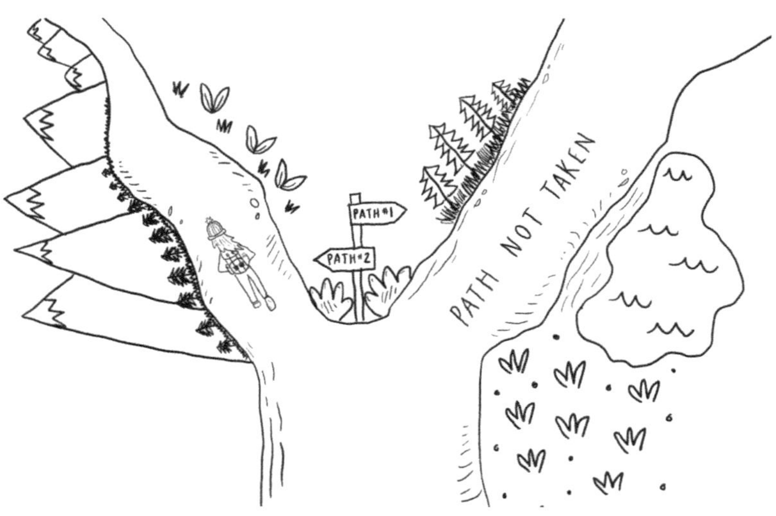

[ 40 ]

# ANYWHERE BUT HERE

July 1st

I've done this tree rings exercise quite a few times by now. But today, it hit different.

Usually, I enjoy it. It typically provides clarity in helpful ways. Everything ends up on one page and I can see all three elements (current, future, blocks) at the same time.

This morning, I became an angsty and annoyed teenager. I found myself spacing out, rolling my eyes, and wanting to be anywhere else.

Instead of just focusing on my business, I made my rings with my entire life in mind.

Because I could feel the temptation to

attribute (or maybe misattribute?) everything that's "not working" to such a major career and identity change.

But I don't tend to enter just one bardo at a time. I'm also going through massive death and rebirth cycles in my personal life and in almost all of my closest relationships.

Trying to look at it all again now... it feels like too much.

I need a break.

I'm going on a hike... hopefully, after that, I'll be able to come back and form thoughts and sentences that actually make sense.

## [ 41 ]
# COSMIC TREE RINGS (CONT.)

Okay... let's try this again, now that I have a little more clarity and my inner teenager isn't so loud...

---

Entrepreneurship is one of the biggest portals to personal growth work. Each stage of entrepreneurship is a ripe opportunity to meet new parts of yourself. Even the parts you don't *want* to meet.

I haven't found a way to skip the personal growth. When done to their fullest potential, both therapy and entrepreneurship transform you. But with any meaningful metamorphosis, there is a "goo" stage of the chrysalis to contend with.

The personal and professional lines are blurred when your life is your business. It's hard to separate out how changes in my relationships are impacting my business. And how career identity shifts are colliding in my personal life.

Part of my exploration this morning led to expected places. Family and friendship dynamics and how all these changes are contributing to an overall sense of feeling unsettled in life.

But as I dug deeper into the middle ring, new clarity emerged about what is *truly* blocking me from the life I desire in the outer ring.

For a long time now, I've been minimizing and trying to hide an aspect of myself.

The part of me that is... (*gasp*)... ***ambitious.***

The part of me that has big and audacious dreams. The part of me that wants to listen to my soul whisper inside, even when she sounds "crazy". That part of me that wants to take a leap into the mystery and trust myself to figure it out. **The part of me that wants to publish powerful books** - *wait, did I really just say that?* The part of me that doesn't want to choose between my work and my family. The part of me that wants to expand and live a big life.

Connecting to my ambition today, I realized something.

I've been apologizing for my ambition because I don't want to make anyone feel bad.

I've been believing an old story that if I fully embrace my ambitious parts, it will hurt other people. *And other people's needs should be prioritized.*

I'm sure I inherited this story from more than one place. Maybe it was being born a girl. Maybe it was my chosen profession as a therapist. Maybe it was from the prevalent societal messages recently villainizing hustle culture. An overcorrection that now glorifies becoming one with your couch - at all times.

Over the past few months, I've already unpacked quite a bit of baggage I was still lugging around from my therapist days. Luggage filled with prescription bottles telling me to water myself down so I don't offend anyone. I've come to understand that my role as someone's therapist was keeping me from becoming the author I wanted to be. But I didn't realize, it went much deeper than that.

**Because what would happen if I just told the truth?**

Well, let's give it a try. The truth is: I have lots of ideas. I want to do lots of things in this life. I want to write books that change people's lives. I want to facilitate transformative retreats. I want to turn *The Self-Trust Model* into a teaching program for therapists and coaches. I want to travel to as many countries as possible and have as many adventures as possible. I want to be the best *Maddy* possible. I want to expand our family and experience the portal of a homebirth. I want to meet myself as a mother. I want to see what an intentional marriage looks like after five decades of the hard work I'm certain will be required of us. I want to sip tea with my bestie inside our witchy teashop. I want to still be summiting mountains when I'm 80. I want to open all the books inside *The Midnight Library*.

- Would people think I was shaming them for wanting something different in life?
- Would people misunderstand my ambition for the way I think everyone should do life?
- Would people accuse me of being a victim of capitalism?

Fear tells me the answer to all of these questions is a demonstrable, "Yes".

But, as I go back and re-read the list of me just telling the truth to myself, something is abundantly clear to me. Not a single one of the things I mentioned is a *Life-Script* someone told me to do. *Except being a mother - but they were only telling me that when I was in my twenties. And the way I want to experience it now, is lightyears from any script I was handed back then.*

**All the wild ambitions I have in life are mine.** The desire for those things comes from within. Not from feeling like I "should".

And that's the entire essence of *The Self-Trust Model* at its core.

It's not giving you a prescription for a good life. It's giving you a framework and tools to discover it for yourself. If I really believe in the model, I can trust that people will discover that for themselves. They can see me embracing my natural ambition and not take it on as "The One True Path".

It is actually respectful of people's sovereignty, to assume they're capable of seeing the nuance. Witnessing me embrace a part of myself doesn't mean they have to have the exact same part in themselves. But maybe, they can be inspired to embrace their own parts. Even if the part they want to get to know, looks nothing like ambition.

> What does this mean for my business and my personal life?
>
> How would my ambitious part want to show up if she wasn't so afraid of her presence hurting someone else?

These are questions I'm really excited to discover the answers to.

After you've completed this exercise, I encourage you to take a moment to reflect on the process.

**How was it for you?**

What I've noticed in doing this exercise with many women, is that you don't always get clarity on the outer ring right away. Sometimes it's hard to identify what your hopes, dreams, and the life you desire really is.

Sometimes, you first get clarity on what you *don't* want.

You might have a clear sense of *"not this"*, but don't yet know what you do want.

This is when Self-Trust is critical. Because it takes courage and trust to say *'No'* to something without yet knowing what you want to say *'Yes'* to.

I experienced this when I received the clarity that it was time to end my therapy practice. The *'No'* in my body and soul was clear. Crystal clear. But I didn't yet have access to what I would do *instead* of running a private practice full time.

Thankfully, I'd had enough reps by that point to know what was required of me. I would have to take the leap if I wanted what was possible on the other side.

But it wasn't a leap of faith.

**It was a leap of trust.**

Faith is an unearned version of trust.

And because of the trust I've cultivated in myself, I knew it would make sense... eventually. I knew, at some point in the future, I'd be able to connect the dots. But if I waited to take action until I had all the logical information, it wouldn't be possible.

When I got the clear message to end my practice, I didn't have access yet to the things that would make the decision make sense. It wasn't until I listened and took action, that I was able to see the reasons why it was necessary.

So, if as you filled out your rings, you weren't able to clearly articulate what you desire in the outer ring, that's okay! Notice if you got access to your *"not this"*. That's enough information to begin.

This exercise gets to grow and evolve with you. This is when the practice begins to look like tree rings.

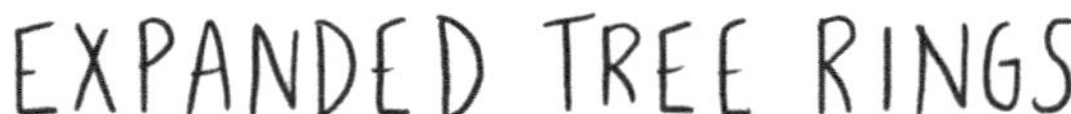


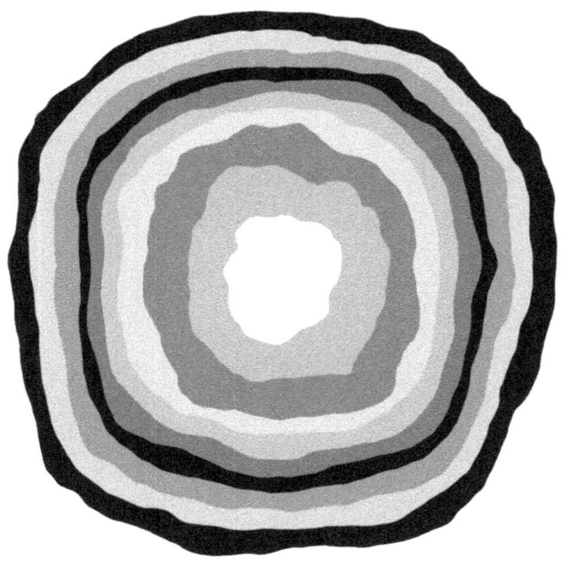

You have the option in life to continue to expand and change. You can reinvent yourself as many times as you want. **The outer ring you filled out today with your aspira-**

**tions and goals, could one day be the inner ring - your starting point.** And when you identify the next round of hopes and dreams, you'll discover a new ring of fears and blocks as well.

In the business world, I often hear the phrase, "*New levels, new devils.*"

If you're like me, the process of expanding into the next ring is exciting. Even if it comes with new devils. I enjoy thinking about what comes next and what it will take to get there (*Oh hey there, ambition*). The more challenging aspect for me, is welcoming the necessary contraction. But both are required. It's how our nervous system works. **Allowing the natural rhythm and flow of the expansion and contraction cycles are how we build more capacity in our nervous system.** You can't be in a constant state of expansion.

The growth edge for many of us, is to actually *be* in the outer ring for a while once you get there. It's taking time to slow down and be present with yourself and your people in the outer ring you worked so hard to get to. **The imperative role of integration.**

I know this concept well. I preach this concept. And, it's still so hard for me to actually do.

A few days ago, the group program I was running came to an end. We focused most of the final call on prioritizing time to reflect on progress, celebrate each other's wins, and bring intention to closing our group time together. I'm good at reminding other people how important this part is.

Immediately when I woke up the next morning, my brain was already onto "*What's next?*"

I had to very deliberately slow down and set time in my calendar to reflect on the beta round of the program. Because I know how important it is.

Thankfully, *Past Me* also knew my tendencies.

At the beginning of the year, my husband and I went through the calendar and scheduled celebration nights after "wins" in our business. So there was already a dim sum + ice cream celebration on the calendar for the following evening.

One final thing to consider when you look at the rings you create.

To get from the inside ring to the outer ring, you have to go through the "hard" of the middle ring. You have to navigate through the fears and the blocks.

But choosing to stay contained in the inside ring is a different kind of hard.

**Choose your hard.**

# [ 42 ]
# EAST: KEEP PROMISES

**How do you learn you can trust someone?**

They do what they say they are going to do.

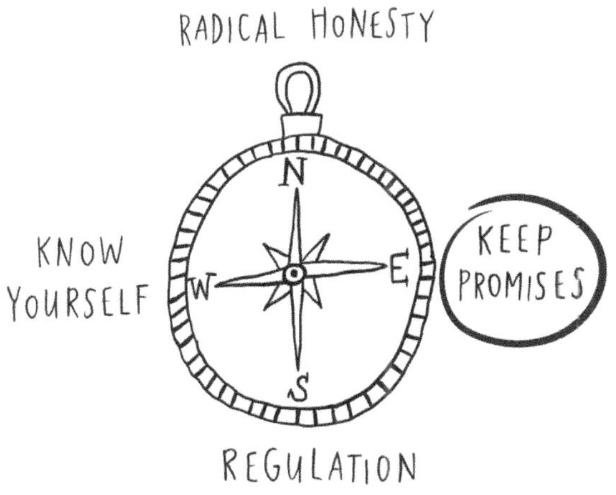

Exactly. The simplest path to trusting yourself is becoming a trustworthy person. And trustworthy people follow through on their commitments. They keep their promises.

The same applies to building trust with yourself. If you want to trust yourself more, following through is a requirement. When you habitually follow through on your commitments, it eventually gets to the point when you almost have no choice *but* to trust yourself. But trust doesn't happen overnight. Consistency over time is what allows trust to build from within.

This is super simple... as a concept.

> *"Just do what you say you're going to do."*

But, it's not that easy for most people. In fact, East is the direction I hear the most pushback and resistance from people when they initially learn about the compass. Often for many good reasons.

And then, notice what happens when I tell you it's also about keeping the "right" promises. Stick with me...

**If we over-simplify what I've seen, people often fall into two categories:**

- People who come up with lots of "good reasons" to not follow through.
- People who *always* follow through on *every* promise, but are still struggling to trust themselves.

Since these two categories are essentially at opposite ends of the spectrum, the growth edges will be different. It's helpful if you first identify which category you most often fit into.

**We'll start with those of you who have every justification for why "this time" it makes sense to *not* follow through.**

First off, I'm totally okay if my assertion that you have to follow through on your commitments to trust yourself, is completely false. I'm ready for you to prove me wrong! Actually, I bet you could make a lot of people happy with that discovery too. So...

- Keep flaking on yourself.
- Don't follow through.
- Break promises to yourself.
- Don't hold the line with your boundaries.

And if you find that you're able to trust yourself. Let me know! That would be a really relieving revelation for many people.

---

But, if you're ready to follow the compass and build the Self-Trust muscle, I encourage you to start small. Just like if you were to begin a new weightlifting routine. Don't try to max out the first day. You'll probably pull a muscle and not return to the gym for a year.

I love the way I've heard *Julie Jeske* speak about trust. I'm pretty sure she was speaking about trust in a relationship with someone else, but it applies to Self-Trust too.

> *"Trust is less like a light switch that you turn on or off, and more like 100 candles that you light (or blow out) one at a time."*

Start small. With the tiniest promise you could make to yourself. Follow through on it. Then do it again tomorrow. And the next day. Then commit to doing it for a week. A month...

You get the point.

Each time you keep a promise to yourself, it's a rep in the right direction. Once it becomes a habit for you to follow through, it would be silly to *not* trust yourself to do it.

Keeping promises also applies to holding the line on boundaries you set. Boundaries with yourself and with others. From this perspective it's less about the specific boundary that you set and more about the commitment you make to yourself by setting the boundary.

This is why I really encourage people to *wait* to set a boundary, until they are ready to *actually* follow through on it. Because if you think it's a boundary you're "supposed" to set, but you're not actually ready to hold the line with it, you're setting yourself up to erode any trust you do have.

---

**People struggling to follow through, let's get practical with your To-Do List for a bit.**

First, I invite you to explore the paradoxical space of these two questions:

- *How can I approach my To-Do list as a way to follow through on my commitments to myself that will ultimately lead to more Self-Trust?*

- *How do I not attach my worth to the completion of my To-Do list tasks?*

Next, let's explore your current relationship with your To-Do list:

- *Is it a friendly and helpful companion? Encouraging you and cheering you on?*
- *Is it a practical confidant? A judgment-free space to get everything out of your head?*
- *Is it a taunting critic? Always reminding you where you're falling short?*

Take a moment and get radically honest about how you're approaching your To-Do list.

- *What's already working?*
- *What's not?*

All the answers to these questions are going to help you to decide how much tweaking you'll need with your To-Do list.

*Warning:* I'm about about to offer you a bunch of ideas to try out and see if they help you with following through. But there's a good chance you don't need all of them. Maybe start by skimming the ideas and try out just one or two. You can always come back and try the others later.

*Ideas to Revamp Your To-Do List:*

## Reflective To-Do List

- Identify a goal you have - maybe one of the things you wrote down in the outer ring of your *Cosmic Tree Rings.*
- What have you already done over the past three months to get you closer to the goal?

- Write out every single thing you've already done.
- Then, one by one - cross them all off your list.
- Feel the dopamine hit. Give yourself credit and celebrate your progress!
- Ride the wave of momentum towards your goals.

## Connect to Your Future Self

Earlier in this book, we explored how following through on a commitment to yourself can be something your *Future Self* will thank you for.

I once received a "Note from the Universe" email that said:

*"Enjoying short-term pleasures at the expense of long-term dreams is just as silly as pursuing long-term dreams at the expense of short-term pleasures. Pursue both."*

I remember this when I'm considering my goals, intentions, and To-Do list tasks. What promises do I want to make to myself that considers both my versions of me? My *Present Self* and my *Future Self*.

Because life is happening in this exact moment. *This* moment is my life. I want to be present and enjoy it. *And* I know that how I live today and the goals I set now, impact how I get to live in the future.

## Get Curious

If you're struggling to check off an item on your To-Do List, I really want to encourage you to slow down and get curious about why. Sometimes it's just because the item is too big. **Not everything has to be rooted in childhood trauma and require a decade of therapy!** If it's just too big, break it down into smaller chunks and try again.

Sometimes though, there are deeper reasons why we're not able to follow through on commitments. When this happens, get really curious about all the different parts of you.

**Ask yourself:**

- *Which part of you made this commitment?*
- *Who added this task to your to-do list?*
- *Was it you?*
- *Or was it "Should"?*

There's a reason most New Year's resolutions aren't kept. And why many people adopt the narrative that they "can't follow through". *Life-Scripts* come into play again and all the ways we're told what our goals "should" be.

Only following what you think you "should" do and making commitments to yourself from that place, often sets you up for failure. Instead, I encourage you to think about the intention underneath the commitment. What is it that *you* really want when you set a goal to "lose 10lbs", "take a trip to Europe", or "quit your job"?

When you slow down and connect to what *you* really desire in life, you're able to set goals and intentions that are more aligned. And this gives you a much better chance of following through.

### Identify "Self-Sabotage"

Sometimes, it looks like self-sabotage when you're not able to get through the things on your To-Do list. Here are some things to consider if you're able to identify "the one thing" that you can't seem to cross off. The one that always gets pushed to the next day.

Notice how you feel towards the part of you that is blocking you from completing the task. (*It's really difficult to learn more about the part if you're feeling angry or annoyed with it. Try to access curiosity and understanding to genuinely want to learn about this part.*)

- How familiar is this part?
- How often does it show up in your life?
- Does it show up in other areas of your life?

What is this part afraid would happen if it stopped doing its job? (Its job = not letting you complete the task you want to do.)

Here are some things you might notice arise when you slow down and get curious about this part... See if any of these resonate with you.

- This task is connected to an internalized *Life-Script* (as explored above)
- You're afraid of whatever comes AFTER completing this task.
    - Ex. Responsibility that comes with success, having to "justify" success, etc.
- You're overwhelmed and your nervous system is in a freeze state.
- Realistically, you're just not able to prioritize this item in your life right now.

## Radical Honesty

This is another opportunity for *Radical Honesty*. Be honest with yourself about the season of life that you're currently in. Because some seasons of life are meant for expansion and hustle and exponential growth and fun! Other times, you'll find yourself in a season of survival. When the best goal you can set for yourself is to just make it through the day.

- Be honest with yourself about the season of life you're *actually* in, not the season you *wish* you were in.
- Set goals from this honest place, not from the goals you see other people setting.

### Rest + Enjoy

Remember to give yourself credit when you do reach your goals. This is one of the more challenging things for me to put into practice, but it's incredibly valuable. When you do check something off your To-Do list or reach a goal:

- Can you let yourself celebrate and enjoy your efforts?
- Can you give yourself credit for all the small wins along the way that contributed to you becoming the person you want to be?

Adding in this piece really allows you to re-write any narratives you may have that you're just a "person who doesn't follow through." This is a chance to show yourself the evidence that you *can and do* keep your promises. You *can and do* follow through. And each time you pause and notice it when it happens, it's building up the embodied knowing that you can be trusted when you say you're going to do something.

---

**Now, let's shift to people on the other end of the spectrum.**

**People who *always* follow through on *every* promise, but are still struggling to trust themselves.**

There's nuance to consider when keeping promises. Just because you follow through on every single commitment you set without fail, it doesn't mean that you'll have unwavering Self-Trust.

**You have to make sure you're setting and keeping the "right" promises.**

Sometimes, you actually have to *break* a promise, in order to come back in integrity with yourself and your values. So, in fact, it's not *always* flaky to break a promise. Breaking a promise doesn't automatically mean you become less trustworthy.

*Hear me out...*

If you make a commitment from the part of you that is a bit of a people-pleaser, you might not actually *want* to follow through. But you do it anyway. This part might be prioritizing someone else's feelings above your own.

If you make a commitment from a Competitive or Perfectionist Part of you, she might be prioritizing a *Life-Script* over what is actually aligned with your life and values.

When you make and follow through on commitments that aren't in integrity with who you are, you don't actually cultivate more Self-Trust. In fact, it can have the opposite effect. You may disconnect so much from yourself, that you actually *lose* trust in yourself.

There's also the element of the sunk cost fallacy to consider. This is the tendency to continue pouring time, money, and energy into a goal - simply because you've already committed to it. Even after you discover the goal no longer makes sense or it's out of integrity. Continuing on the path based on commitment bias.

It's the rationale of, *"But, I've already spent thousands upon thousands of dollars and years of my life to get my degree, I have to keep a job in this field."*

Sometimes, the best thing you can do for yourself - is quit.

If this resonates with you, your growth edge might actually be to *break* a commitment you set. You may need to course correct and pivot on the promises you've made to yourself.

**Discernment is powerful here - knowing when to follow through, and when to pivot.**

Moving forward, the most important thing you can do is set the "right" promises. These are the promises made from your wise and competent Self energy. You want to make promises to yourself that are aligned with *your* values, not with the unexamined *Life-Scripts*. This sets you up for success and more ease in following through.

When you make promises to yourself from Self energy and alignment with your values, it's less likely that you'll have other parts come in and self-sabotage.

---

**Regardless of if you always follow through or struggle to keep promises to yourself, this final piece can be helpful for both.**

Find a way to add "completion" to the promise you made, even if it wasn't "met" in the way you anticipated. This can relieve the burden of carrying a narrative that *"I can't trust myself to follow through"*.

This might be breaking a promise to come back into integrity with your values. Or pivoting on the goal once you have more information about the direction you're headed. Discernment of when to follow through and when to pivot - can be your superpower. And, in my opinion, it's right up there with flying.

[ 43 ]

# MANTRAS FOR KEEPING PROMISES:

- I will follow through on my commitments.
- I will hold the line on the boundaries I set; especially when it's uncomfortable.
- I will follow through until I have no choice but to trust myself.

[ 44 ]

## MANTRAS FOR BREAKING PROMISES:

- I will pivot on promises not made from my wisest Self.
- I will keep only the "right" promises to myself.
- I will break a promise to myself if that's what's required to trust myself more.

# [ 45 ]
# A WRITER

The earlier chapter on ambition might give you a hint as to where I personally tend to land on the spectrum of keeping promises. Following through on what I say I'm going to do is my comfort zone.

Sometimes to a fault.

So, I've had to learn when the right answer is actually to intentionally break a commitment in order to come back into integrity. Even when it hurts someone's feelings. Ending a marriage. Ending a therapeutic relationship. Stop running marathons with a torn meniscus. *Thankfully, I don't think that last one hurt anybody's feelings though.*

I've become more intentional and clear in what I'm *actually* committing to when I make a promise. To myself or someone else. I want to really understand the intention underneath the goal I have, and set commitments connected to the essence of the intention. I'm striving to make promises from my Self energy as much as possible.

So, when my individual therapy practice was done, I entertained a thousand ideas about what could be next. Primarily focusing on what could be the obvious next step and also the thing that had been lighting me up for a while: facilitating retreats and other group work. Each potential idea came with a long checklist of tactical steps to implement. Which was really at odds with my desire to work *less* and have more time for family. But still, I tried to make it all work. I was mediocrely doing a hundred things.

Thankfully, I didn't have to hit rock bottom this time in order to get radically honest with myself. Several weeks of low level burnout was enough to catalyze me into change.

**It was clear I needed to pivot on my business goals for the year.**

In hindsight, the unusual-for-me commitment to slow down many of the ideas and projects swirling in my head was a defining moment. That's when I made the uncomfortable commitment to focus on one primary project for the next three months - "The 13 Lessons".

Unfortunately for me, the one project I committed to had no immediate financial return. In my therapy practice, I was accustomed to a tight feedback loop. Have a session with a client and immediately get paid.

*This* was not going to be *that*. Even if the writing is good.

Focusing my attention on a blog series about the lessons I learned as a therapist wasn't going to replace my old income. But I knew it was the next right step. It was clear to me that my focus needed to be on sharing *this* particular writing. Trusting that I'd be able to connect the dots eventually, *if* I listened and took action now.

This commitment was asking me to surrender. Not "fake surrender". I couldn't self-soothe by creating a quick program to fill the void and make some money. True surrender was allowing the void to be there, as long as it was necessary.

So I did it. I put other ideas on hold. I told myself I'd keep the current offerings running, but not start anything new. I'd focus my time primarily on "The 13 Lessons" and whatever it was meant to become.

**So... wait...**

- *Did I just become a writer?*
- *Did I need a permission slip from someone?*

I've spent the past few years adamantly stating that I'm *not* a writer (*while spending thousands of hours writing*). Now, am I supposed to tell people I *am* a writer? I'm not sure I'm ready for that. But that's kinda the reality of what my days look like now.

[ 46 ]

# THAT'S ENOUGH FOR NOW

July 27th

This is the work I came here to do.

I can no longer silence the calls from the universe...

From my soul...

From the reason I'm meant to be here.

I'm doing the work I came here to do.

Even though most days I don't "get it".

My soul gets it.

My body gets it.

And that's enough for now.

## [ 47 ]

## "YOU NEED TO LEAVE YOUR MARRIAGE"

Making steadfast and confident decisions connected to your deepest inner wisdom might be one of the greatest aspirations you can have, if you want to live a meaningful life you love.

It shouldn't come as a surprise given the title of this book and the stories I've shared so far, that I *do* desire to live a life I love. I'm also aware by this point, that making steadfast and confident decisions won't always be easy. And the decisions won't always be what my ego *wants* the answer to be.

The story of my first marriage is better left for a different book. But the cliff notes version is - he was my best friend. My college sweetheart. My favorite person in the world. We had thirteen years of fun memories together. We were good at compromise and didn't really fight that much.

He had agreed when we eloped to take a yearly anniversary trip because I love traveling. We'd been to Ireland, Italy, Iceland. And that first year - when money was tight - Iowa.

That seventh and final year we celebrated, we'd broken away from the "I" locations, and were off to explore the San Juan Islands off the coast of Washington.

It was on this late fall hike that my body started talking to me. Or rather, when I finally started listening to her. In reflection I can now see some attempts at communication leading up to the trip. And maybe even a slight echo of her trying to get my attention a couple of months before the trip. But I hadn't been ready to listen.

Instead, I kept following what made logical sense. And that's how we ended up on the hike combining so many of my favorite things - outdoor adventure, travel, and my best friend. But my stomach... was nauseous.

The urge to vomit kept distracting me from the magical and foggy views synonymous with the Pacific Northwest. With each step, my stomach became more uneasy and I began replaying what I'd eaten. Trying to find the culprit. Maybe it was the first meal we'd had when we arrived. The three-inch french toast I'd been dreaming about ever since my first trip to Seattle two years before. But no, that's not possible. I'd only been able to eat a few bites.

*That's weird. I never lose my appetite.* And super disappointing as I'm always trying to recreate my favorite travel meals. But I'd been dreaming about this trip for months and I wanted to enjoy it.

*"Be. Here. Now."* became my mantra with each step in the forest. But I couldn't. Not fully. My body kept distracting me. Kept tugging at my attention. Back to the nausea.

It was clear my body was trying to tell me something, but I wasn't fully fluent in her native tongue. The line of communication to my physical vessel was still relatively new. After decades of disconnection from my body, it has been a long and slow process to hear her again. And many messages still got lost in translation.

I continued a few more miles, trying to gaslight my body into believing that everything was in fact - "Fine". But damn, she was stubborn. And eventually she ups the ante. She bypasses the body cues all together and delivers a clear message. Straight to (*or rather from*) - my soul.

**"You need to leave your marriage."**

*Excuse me, what?!*

Talk about a blindside. *No, no, body - you don't understand.* At that moment, I turned around and saw my favorite person. Walking on the trail behind me, smiling. He was hiking because *I* love hiking.

I immediately think this is some kind of miscommunication. I probably misheard her.

**"You need to leave your marriage."**

Fuuuck, she seems pretty clear. But she's probably confused. She's probably thinking about OTHER people's relationships. There are a lot of people that shouldn't be together. People that constantly fight and hurt each other. But that wasn't us. I loved him. And he loved me - unconditionally. And in ways I'd never experienced before. Plus, I really *liked* him. Which from what I've seen, is even more rare. Day to day life is easy. And fine. He's your favorite roommate you've ever had. He's stable and solid. He's kind.

*Is she listening? Is the bargaining working?*

**"You need to leave your marriage."**

Oh no… the nausea again. The bargaining might be making it worse. She's not responding to logic or reason. She's not listening to his wonderful attributes. It's almost as if she doesn't care how good of a man he is. Or how much everyone else loves him. Or how much this would hurt him. It's almost as if prioritizing *his* feelings isn't *her* biggest concern.

But what about *my* feelings? Doesn't she see me freaking out? Doesn't she understand that leaving my best friend and the life we've built together would wreck me? Doesn't she understand that what she's telling me to do is impossible?

The self-righteous inner dialogue continues… Who the fuck does she think she is? Telling *me* what to do with *my* life?

And with that, she decides to formally introduce herself to me…

**"Hey, it's me, your intuition."**

---

That's clearly not the end of the story. It was just the beginning of a painful year that could've been considered one of my first "blow it all up" seasons of life. All along, I was holding onto hope that by taking everything apart, I'd eventually be able to put it back together in ways that made more sense.

- *What did you notice as you read about my experience in deciding to leave my marriage?*
- *Did your body respond with recognition - as so many women who've also ended relationships have told me it did?*
- *Did my inner message feel prescriptive to you?*

I encourage you to just sit with your reaction for a while. Notice what you notice. And when you're ready, I have another story to share. Another time my intuition was as clear as she was inconvenient.

---

**"Should I stay? Or should I go?"**

This is a question I've heard countless times from my therapist chair.

I always knew that *their* answer to that question wasn't in me. And they knew it too. Deep down. But knowing that it was their decision to make, didn't stop their penetrating stares from piercing my heart, pleading with me to help "save" them from having to decide.

I could see their desire for someone (*anyone!*) to swoop in and reassure them that they didn't have to do whatever the scary thing they knew they needed to do was.

Sometimes, trusting yourself looks like the big "blow up your life" kind of changes.

Sometimes, the most inconvenient truth is: **you need to go.**

But not always.

Sometimes, the most inconvenient truth is: **you need to stay.**

Maybe... trusting yourself will lead you to meditating alone at an ashram for six months. Or years of nomadic living - sometimes in a tent. Or building a new life from scratch.

Or maybe... trusting yourself will lead you to showing up for hours-long difficult conversations as you navigate hard times and the complexity of doing life intentionally with another complex human.

As hard as leaving my first marriage was (*and I'm not sugar coating it - it fucking sucked*), the discomfort of the "Go" message is still easier for me than the discomfort of the "Stay" message.

Having a *"life will never be the same"* hit of intuition and then digging myself out of the rubble left behind is my discomfort - comfort zone. If I *have* to be uncomfortable, I'm much more comfortable with the option that includes running. And starting over. Preferably in a new zip code.

But that's not always the answer I've received from my inner compass.

Years after the decision to leave my marriage, I was once again confronted with an inconvenient truth.

This time, with a different answer.

This time, I was in a fundamentally different relationship. A relationship that started with two grown adults who had lived a lot of life before meeting each other. Two grown adults with no plans of doing life together forever. But as time went on, slowly came to the realization together that what was happening between the two of them - was worth jumping in with both feet. To give this indescribable and undeniable connection a real shot.

As I hope I've shown you so far, choosing to live a deliberate and intentional life, connected to your values and integrity, actively addressing your blocks and past pain - is not necessarily an easy path. As any worthwhile path is, it can be rife with challenges.

Now, add in doing life like this - *WITH ANOTHER PERSON*. Another person who has their own set of blocks and past pain. A different set of life experiences that have shaped their values. Their own set of wounds that butt right up against your wounds - poking each other.

**Here's the question I had to sit with:**

*Can I trust myself to 'Stay' as much as I trust myself to 'Go'?*

I'd had enough experience to know that I could trust myself to leave a relationship (or job or other situation) that wasn't best for either of us. But could I trust myself to stay in a relationship that *was* pushing me to be the best version of myself?

My protective parts wanted to keep me from getting hurt again. One way to do that is to build walls up around your heart. So I tried that - along with an electric fence. And some well placed snipers. My protective parts reminded me how liberating it feels to run free - not having to answer to anyone. They reminded me that the plan was never to stay. They reminded me that love doesn't last. They reminded me that people die. They tried to entice me with foreign cities I could live in - alone. They reminded me that love makes you vulnerable - and I needed a break from heartbreak.

All the rational reasons to run.

All the logical reasons to go.

But once again, it's as if my intuition doesn't even care what Reason and Logic have to say. Over and over again, each time I'd get spooked in this new relationship, I'd check in with my body and soul.

And each and every time, the answer was annoyingly simple: **"Stay."**

---

That's clearly not the end of this story either. It was just the beginning of a lifetime of big and magical love. Filled with equal amounts of contraction and expansion. A lifetime of putting my life together in ways that make more sense.

- *What did you notice as you read about my experience to stay in a relationship?*
- *Did your body respond with recognition as so many women who've been more comfortable being hyper-independent have told me it did?*
- *Did my inner message feel prescriptive to you?*

I encourage you to just sit with your reaction for a while. Notice what you notice.

**Sometimes, the scary and right thing to do is to go.**

**Sometimes, the scary and right thing to do is to stay.**

## [ 48 ]
# SUPERPOWERS

Building strong discernment muscles is at the core of cultivating more trust in yourself.

> **Discernment is the ability to perceive, understand, and judge things clearly. Especially when things aren't obvious or straightforward.**

We already explored how discernment comes into play when keeping promises. Building the muscles of discernment helps you to know when to follow through on a commitment you set and when the answer is to pivot. That's powerful. But there's even more possibility when you hone your discernment skills.

**Discernment truly becomes your right-up-there-with-flying superpower when you're able to discern between**:

- Intuition and *Life-Scripts*
- Intuition and Anxiety
- Intuition and Wishful Thinking

Okay, you might be noticing a theme with discernment and Self-Trust. This "intuition" word keeps coming up. You received a formal introduction from *my* intuition in the previous chapter, but what does this word actually mean?

As important as I think definitions are, I often struggle to define "intuition". It's the same way I struggle to put words to an experience Mama Shroom offers me. The ineffability of it, is part of what defines it. But I'm going to give it my best shot to define what I mean when I use the word *intuition*. Because, I know when I hear people use the word, we're not always talking about the same thing.

**Here are a few phrases I've used to describe intuition:**

- A soul nudge or pull...
- Deep inner knowing...
- The whisper only I can hear...
- Wisdom that transcends logic...

My intuition comes through as a deep "Knowing" with the utmost clarity. The presence of intuition is steady and unwavering. It's distinct from other thoughts that enter my mind. It has an otherworldly feel to it.

The physical body is the conduit to the metaphysical experience I just described. There is a strong "felt sense" aspect of intuition. Intuition communicates through body sensations. Just as the phrase "*Trust Your Gut*" suggests. This is why I'll often talk about how disconnection from the physical body is also disconnection from intuition. It's like leaving the phone off the hook - calls aren't able to come through. Hmmm... *Does that metaphor even land for people born after 1992?*

Our other senses can also be conduits. You might experience your connection to intuition through sight, sounds, or smells. So much of this work is getting to know the specific and unique way *your* intuition communicates. It takes repetition, patience, and curiosity.

When I'm able to listen to my intuition, I know I'm on a path that is necessary for me to explore. It does *not* mean that it will always be the "Right" path - just that it's the right path at the right time, for me.

This is a common misconception I hear from people wanting to connect to their intuition and trust themselves more. They have a false belief that using their intuition to guide their decisions will lead them to only joy and pleasure. This expectation can set people up to actually *lose* trust in themselves. Because if following their intuition leads them to pain, friction, or setbacks - they feel their intuition "failed them". They begin to discredit their intuition.

*Fleur Leussink* captures this beautifully in her book, *Moving Beyond*, about intuition and spiritual connection:

> *"An intuitive life is not a life in which you are protected from human experience; quite the opposite. An intuitive life is a life in which you are guided into the most expansive version of yourself."*

Allowing your intuition to be your compass often leads to the *full* range of human experience. Heartbreak. Ecstasy. And everywhere in between.

One more way to capture this comes from South African lion tracker and author, *Boyd Varty*.

> *"As paradoxical as it sounds, going down a path and not finding a track is part of finding the track."*

He goes on to describe the *"Path of Not Here"* as the part of the path to *"Here"*. This is why it's actually possible for the perceived mistakes we make in life to be alchemized to more Self-Trust.

---

Now that you have a better understanding of what I mean when I say intuition, let's come back to discernment as a super-power. Because the differences between:

- Intuition and *Life-Scripts*
- Intuition and Anxiety
- Intuition and Wishful Thinking

... are often subtle. But identifying the differences can be life-changing.

## Intuition and *Life-Scripts*

*Life-Scripts* are often provided to us subconsciously. They become an automatic way of doing life. They feel... familiar. And what we know about the nervous system is that it *likes* things that are familiar.

*In our nervous system:* Familiar = Safe

This is why it can be so challenging to do something new or different. Even when we know the new or different thing is objectively better for us. It's staying with the "devil you know". You know how to navigate and manage the devil you know, so it's more comfortable to stay.

*How this connects to intuition:*

Doing something different in life than how you've been told, will often bring up activation in your system. Your nervous system is put on high alert to scan for threats because you're not operating on autopilot anymore. This necessary activation can come across as a sign that something is wrong and tries to convince you to return to the old way.

One of the strongest *Life-Scripts*, repeatedly handed to me throughout my life, was around motherhood. Even when I politely explained that I didn't want to audition for the role, people kept handing me the script anyways. Family and strangers alike - all seemed to think this was the role I *needed* to play. Mainly, because it's the role *every* woman was supposed to play. Plus, I was happily married to a man who would make an incredible father. There wasn't a single reason why I *shouldn't* drive a minivan down the well paved path ahead of me to a lifetime of backyard barbecues in suburbia.

*Except for the fact that... I didn't want to.*

Except for the fact that every cell in my body screamed *'No'* every time I tried to convince myself with how cute Air Jordan onesies are.

## Intuition and Anxiety

This segues us directly into discerning intuition from anxiety or fear. This is a common dilemma I hear from people. Their body is screaming something at them, but they don't know if it's their intuition telling them not to do something... or anxiety.

It is *really* difficult to trust your intuition when your nervous system is dysregulated. That's why South on the Self-Trust compass is all about nervous system regulation. *More on that to come in a future chapter.*

Access to our intuition often begins by learning the language of the body. Slowing down long enough to connect to the sensations in the physical body and getting curious about the messages being communicated. The practice I encourage people to do starts by asking them a question:

> *"When was the last time you intentionally got out of your comfort zone and did something that scared you?"*

If the answer is some version of *"I don't know..."* or *"Why would I do something like that?"*, then it makes a lot of sense that discerning between anxiety and intuition is hard. Your discernment muscles are weak because they haven't been worked out. It doesn't mean that they aren't there.

The first step I offer to get better at discerning between intuition and anxiety is simple, but often not easy.

*Get uncomfortable. On purpose.*

This practice helps to build up muscle memory about what anxiety feels like in your body when she shows up. Because if you're not familiar with the qualities of anxiety, it's hard to tell the difference between anxiety and inner wisdom.

You want to start by choosing an action step that is aligned with your values, goals, or intentions, but is a little scary when you think about actually doing it. Choose something that is a growth edge for you. It could be an edge in your business. Or maybe you want to get to know anxiety at the edge of a cliff, readying yourself to jump into the water below.

Then, when you do the thing, *really* pay attention. Pay attention to all the ways your body responds, the thoughts that emerge, the emotions, the old beliefs. Notice everything. *You now have an embodied memory of anxiety.* You have something to compare to how your inner wisdom shows up. And the more reps you get, the stronger your discernment muscles become.

Sometimes, you don't even have to go searching for the uncomfortable thing to do. Sometimes, it shows up right in your inbox, in the form of a life changing cease-and-desist letter.

*A little backstory...*

After the idea for the "not-quite-group-therapy" but "not-quite-wellness-retreat" came to me, I wanted to give it a name. As I described the concept to my husband, he commented that it sounded like a book club, but for healing adventures. He was right. But not just any kind of book club. Choice was of the utmost importance. It was a *Choose-Your-Own-Adventure* kind of club. But that's too long of a name.

So it became... *Adventure Club.*

I wanted to create separation from my therapy practice. So I decided to open a second business. Specifically for the non-therapy work I wanted to do. But it needed a name that captured what the offerings would be. I envisioned various pathways to use *The Self-Trust Model*™.

*Adventure Club* would just be one of them. Eventually, there would be lots of choices. Lots of possible adventures. People could choose their own healing adventure. The *Choose Your Own Adventure* coaching business was born.

Fast forward, I discovered the chooseyourownadventure.com domain was available. *Anyone who's ever tried to get a ".com" domain, knows they are worth the few thousand dollar price tag.*

The synchronicities I was experiencing and the loose "legal" advice I obtained was enough for me to feel confident. Until an email with the words "trademark infringement" showed up. But instead of letting anxiety make my decisions, I slowed down. I got into my body. I vetted the advice I was given.

And, I made my decisions moving forward - grounded in my intuition.

These decisions surprisingly did *not* include attorneys or high legal fees. Instead, I asked the CEO of the *Choose Your Own Adventure* book publishing company to get on a video call with me so we could talk through options - options *other* than what was initially written out in the scary email.

This led to multiple negotiation meetings. Each one requiring me to *get uncomfortable; on purpose.* Each time, *almost* allowing anxiety to keep me from showing up. Each one requiring me to advocate for myself in different ways. And each time, strengthening trust with myself.

In the way synchronicities often resemble an onion, the layers to this experience felt infinite. And brought tears to my eyes.

- It began an unexpected mentoring relationship with the same CEO I was initially scared to respond to.
- It led to the surprising realization that it was time to close down my therapy practice.
- It planted a seed about "*one day*" becoming an author.

This experience also prepared me for how loud my anxiety would become over the next few months, trying to talk me out of what my intuition knew to be true.

I hope this example highlights for you that discerning between anxiety and intuition is not as simple as:

Anxiety feels bad. Intuition feels good.

Nothing about this process felt "good" early on. It made me want to throw up most days. And it ultimately led to even more discomfort as I began the process of closing my practice.

But as terrible and scary as it felt most days, I was also tethered to the knowing in my bones... that it was right.

### Intuition and Wishful Thinking

Rounding out your discernment superpowers, I want to focus on the differences between intuition and wishful thinking. Or you might even think of this as rationalization.

I've heard people try to oversimplify the differences between anxiety and intuition by saying that anxiety feels like constriction in your body and intuition feels calm. But as you just read, that's not been my experience. And it's rarely been the case for people I work with. Which is why I also want to include wishful thinking in the conversation around intuition.

And maybe, the best way to illustrate this difference, is with an example.

I had no previous business experience when I started my private practice. My career, up until that point, had been with a variety of different agencies. Most of them offering therapy services for free. I'd accepted that long hours and low pay was my future for the next few decades. Naively thinking I could also avoid burnout and resentment. But, a series of events "nudged" me to leave my agency job. It's possible that the inner whispers had been there for a while, but I'd been plugging my ears, singing *"La, La, La, La, Laaaa"*. The universe got progressively louder, until it was impossible *not* to listen.

So, I went out on my own. Reluctantly starting a private practice, from nothing. Then, I connected with a friend of mine who was a part of a group private practice. A practice where there was already a steady stream of new clients seeking services. The LLC was already created. The tax forms were set up. All the logistics of starting a business - done. The prime location had been secured long ago and the fully furnished office with gorgeous windows awaited me. All I had to do was say "*Yes*" and I could join an established group practice, begin seeing clients immediately, replace my salary, and work with my dear friend. All of this sounded... perfect.

So why when I went to meet the practice owner, did my stomach knot up and my inner wisdom tell me, '*No*', instead?

Confused, I went home and hoped that my intuition was wrong. Maybe she didn't hear all the information about how perfect this opportunity was. Maybe I could sit down and rationally show her the 'Pro List'. Then, she'd have to get it. Logically, everything about this situation made more sense than me going out on my own with zero experience and building up a caseload of clients from scratch. And the timing of it all! It *had* to be a sign that it was the right path.

But, it's almost as if my intuition didn't even care about all the logical and rational reasons I explained to her. Actually, it's *exactly* like she didn't care. Like an unwavering parent who doesn't even take time to justify the '*No*'. My intuition might as well have said, "*Because I said so*" and left it at that.

In hindsight, I understand that there wouldn't have been a way for my intuition to explain to me *why* the answer was no. Even if that was how intuition worked. There's no way I would've understood because I didn't have the information I needed yet.

**I needed to trust the wisdom within even without the logic to back it up.**

Cut to the end. I was able to discern between what my intuition was *actually* telling me and what I wishfully *wanted* the answer to be. Thankfully, I was able to listen to the wisdom that transcends logic and it didn't take long for the reasons to reveal themselves. Less than six months later, clarity came and there hasn't been one day I've regretted taking the seemingly harder path.

[ 49 ]

# THE HANGOVER

August 5th

I wish I would've written in my journal yesterday, because today feels completely different.

Yesterday was the win.

Today... is the hangover.

Vulnerability hangovers are REAL. But I'm trying to remind myself that...

* Today's low doesn't take away from yesterday's high.

* And yesterday's high doesn't take away from today's low.

I'm reassuring myself that the impulse I have to quit everything and move to the forest is an expected part of the process. It doesn't mean I actually have to quit. I'm just experiencing a natural part of the expansion and contraction cycle.

Yesterday was a bright spot after many months of feeling more doubt than confidence.

My fear of "being seen" is still loud. And it might be my biggest block to creating the business I desire. This fear of visibility and vulnerability has been paralyzing in the past. And it won't go away just by pretending it's not there.

I've tried.

Instead, I'm trying something different. And it involves continuing to get uncomfortable... on purpose.

It involves saying "Yes" to interviews and speaking engagements even though the idea of them makes me want to puke.

If I want people to learn about The Self-Trust Model, I have to be willing to talk about it.

Yesterday, I did just that. I recorded a podcast episode (after taking 4 hours beforehand for a final prep).

And even though I was exhausted when we hung up, I was surprised to admit that I actually enjoyed it.

An hour later, another interview I'd said "Yes" to was published and I got to sit and watch (and cringe). Another moment of surprise when I realized it actually wasn't terrible.

A moment of believing I might actually be able to do this.

I'm actively testing the narratives in my head that tell me I can't survive being misunderstood. It still feels existential at times.

Vulnerability and visibility still feel dangerous.

But maybe the idea of "Feel the fear and do it anyways" has some merit.

This is at least a rep in the right direction.

Regardless, all I know is... now I need a nap.

[ 50 ]

# CONVERGENCE

Remember, The *Self-Trust Model*™ exists at the convergence of somatic therapy, "parts work", and psychedelic therapy (with or without medicine).

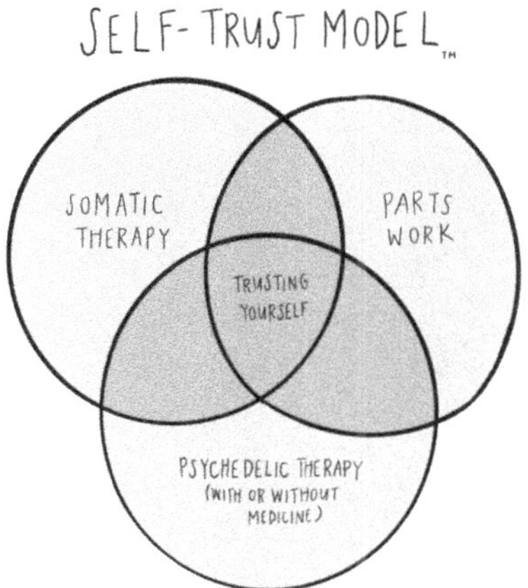


*The Self-Trust Model* wasn't created from the *only* modalities I was trained in. In some ways it formed organically. And yet, it was also intentionally created at the intersections of what I saw to be most effective, personally and professionally. That's not to say there aren't other influences. During my career as a therapist, I had many opportunities to be well-trained in a variety of therapeutic modalities and yoga practices. *I listed them out on page 42.*

So while I focus on the three modalities that primarily make up *The Self-Trust Model*, it would make sense if it is also influenced by the other frameworks. If you're familiar with any of them, you might see their elements woven in as well.

Regardless of what modality I was utilizing, incorporating the physical body into the therapeutic process has been a core foundation of how I have approached my work from the very beginning. A more holistic approach to understanding the mind, body, and spirit connection has always made more sense to me than trying to do any healing in isolation.

Before we continue around the compass to South (Regulation) I want to give you a foundation of nervous system work and somatic therapy, through the lens of *Somatic Experiencing*.

[ 51 ]

# SOMATIC EXPERIENCING® BASICS

"The most important lesson I have gleaned is that we all have the innate capacity to heal."
- Somatic Experiencing developer,
Dr. Peter Levine

*Somatic Experiencing* (SE) is a highly effective body-awareness approach to healing trauma. Stemming from a curiosity about how animals in the wild are routinely threatened existentially, yet they are rarely traumatized.

Humans, with a virtually identical regulatory mechanism, suffer a much different fate.

The human animal is regularly traumatized from not only physical threats, but also threats that are emotional, relational, psychological, existential, and spiritual in nature.

. . .

Us humans are plagued with a myriad of trauma symptoms such as:

- Anxiety
- Depression
- Hypervigilance
- Addiction
- Sexual dysfunction
- Fibromyalgia
- Eating disorders
- Cognitive dysfunction
- Dissociation
- Chronic pain and autoimmune disorders
- Emotion regulation problems
- Phobias

Just to name a few...

Thankfully all animals, humans included, have a nervous system that is capable of returning to stability and balance within. We just have to know how to connect to it and work *with* it. Which most of us were not taught.

*Somatic Experiencing* offers a framework that can be a portal back to our innate capacity to heal.

## Nervous System 101 (and 201)

The Autonomic Nervous System (ANS) is automatic - "auto" - it operates without our control, it regulates all the basic functions of our bodies - including heart rate, breathing, blood pressure, digestion, and more.

It's also the source of our survival responses.

. . .

There are two branches of the ANS:

- Sympathetic Nervous System (SNS)
- Parasympathetic Nervous System (PNS)

| SYMPATHETIC NERVOUS SYSTEM (SNS) | PARASYMPATHETIC NERVOUS SYSTEM (PNS) |
|---|---|
| • ACTS LIKE A GAS PEDAL | • ACTS LIKE A BRAKE PEDAL |
| • MOBILIZING ENERGY TO TAKE ACTION | • HELPS US REST AND RESET |
| • RELEASES ADRENALINE FUELING THE FIGHT OR FLIGHT RESPONSE | • CAN RELEASE NATURAL OPIODS TO REDUCE PAIN -FUELING FREEZE RESPONSE |
| • PREPARES US TO MEET A THREAT | • HELPS US UNWIND AND LET GO OF MUSCLE TENSION |
| • TRAUMA CAN RESULT IN HYPERAROUSAL - CAUSING US TO THINK WE ARE CONSTANTLY UNDER ATTACK. | • TRAUMA CAN RESULT IN CHRONIC HYPOAROUSAL -CAUSING US TO DISCONNECT FROM THE BODY & ACTUAL THREATS |
| 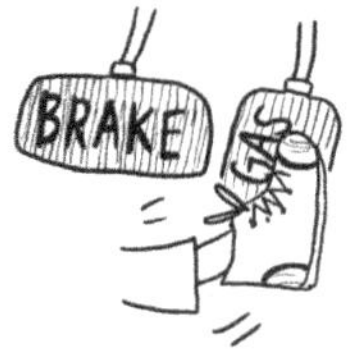 BRAKE GAS | BRAKE GAS |

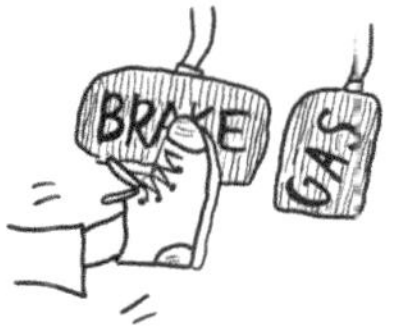

Okay, stay with me, because the PNS is a bit more complicated. But I'm going to simplify it as much as possible. This essential element to understanding our nervous system comes from *Polyvagal Theory*, the work of Dr. Stephen Porges. (*Poly - many; vagal - related to vagus nerve*). The vagus nerve is the longest cranial nerve in the human body. It runs from the brainstem down through all the major organs - and if you have one - into the cervix.

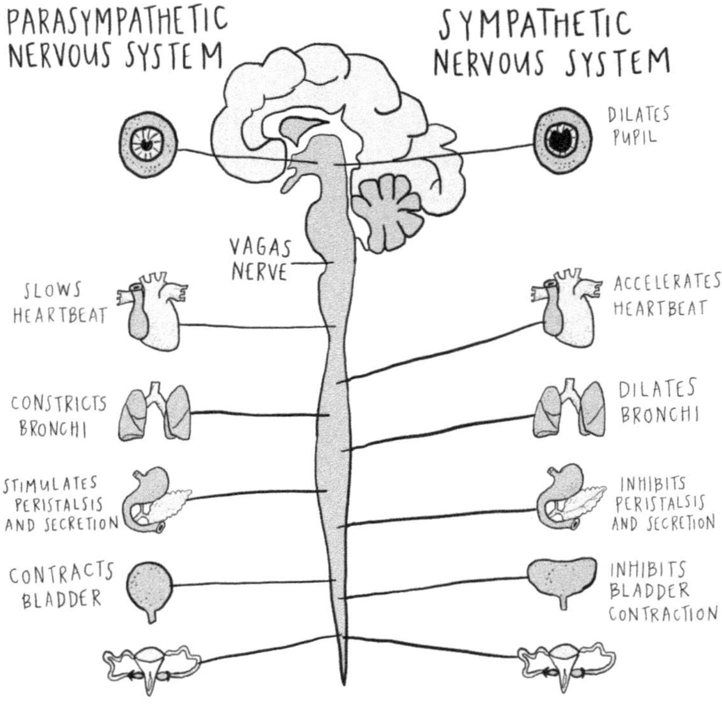


The PNS consists of 2 pathways found in the vagus nerve with very different functions:

- Ventral Vagal Pathway
- Dorsal Vagal Pathway

*Ventral Vagal:*

- Responds to cues of safety and social connection
- This allows for rest, connection, sense of ease, and capacity for healthy relationships.
- Brake pedal

*Dorsal Vagal:*

- Responds to cues of extreme threat
- This triggers our most primitive survival instincts - shutdown, disconnect, feeling frozen, and preparing for death.
- Pulling the emergency handbrake while the gas is still floored

That's why appearing "calm" on the outside is not always indicative of safety and regulation in the nervous system. This helps us understand that these nervous system states are not "good" or "bad". They all serve important functions for survival. The issue is when we get "stuck" in one of these states and can't return to a normal range of regulation.

## Healthy Nervous System Response

The goal of working *with* the nervous system is not to try and achieve an eternal mythical zen state of chanting "om" on the mountaintop. I for one, would be very bored with a flatline existence, perpetually trapped in a state of "regulation".

A healthy nervous system mimics other aspects of nature with cycles of expansion and contraction. Cycles of charge and discharge. When healthy and under threat, your nervous system can identify the threat and respond appropriately. It will either:

- Activate: Fight or Flight (increased arousal in SNS)
- Or: Freeze (increased arousal in dorsal vagal part of PNS)

Once the threat is gone, a healthy nervous system is able to discharge the survival energy (fight/flight/freeze) and return to the ventral vagal part of the PNS. This is when you're able to feel relaxed and at ease. You're able to feel settled and safe again.

**The capacity to move into states of activation when necessary and then return back to a settled state is the hallmark of a healthy nervous system.**

When you have health and vitality in your nervous system it supports Self-Trust because you trust yourself to respond appropriately to threats when they arise.

A practice you can do to get to know your nervous system better is to graph it.

- What does your nervous system graph look like from the past 24 hours?
- What does your nervous system graph look like on a typical day? Week?

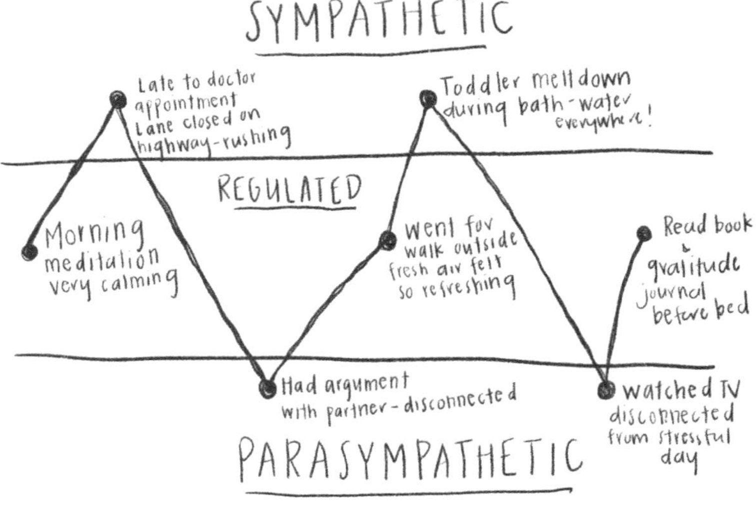

*Side note:* Increased arousal in the SNS is not "bad" and it's not just the fight or flight response we think of when we're under perceived threat. Activation in the SNS can also occur in a healthy nervous system during times of excitement and fun, during sexual activity, and can be a mobilizing agent for positive change in your life.

## Trauma

We've been talking a lot about how trauma impacts the nervous system. Let's revisit the definition of trauma we're using for the purpose of this book.

Trauma: *anything* that overwhelms your nervous system's ability to cope *can be* registered as traumatic. Anything that is too much, too soon, or too fast. It's not about the specific event itself. It's about the impact on the nervous system, which includes the support you receive afterwards. *Or, lack thereof.*

When your nervous system is overwhelmed, it goes into survival mode. This means the survival energy of the fight, flight, freeze response gets activated. And if the survival energy doesn't have a chance to move through and be discharged from your body, it can get "stuck" in your system.

*What sensations do you notice in your body as you hear "trauma" described?*

Do you notice any of the following:

- Shaky
- Sweaty
- Buzzy
- Floaty
- Twitchy
- *Something else?*

**Want more? Here's a longer list of to help build your vocabulary for Language of Sensation.**

Noticing how your body and nervous system responds to words, people, experiences, and ideas is a first step to strengthening your relationship with yourself and supporting a healthy nervous system.

Once you identify a sensation in your body, try to be with it for a moment. Just notice it.

And then, you can ask yourself the question that used to make me sound like a broken record in sessions:

> **"And then what happens?"**

"Tracking Your Sensations" does not come naturally for many people and requires intentional practice. It's a powerful practice of continually following what you notice happening in your body. It allows us to explore the "body story" instead of just the cognitive story:

- Does the sensation change when you pay attention to it?
- Does it decrease or increase?
- Does it move or stay in the same place?

- Does it shift to a different kind of sensation?
- Does it go away completely?
- Does it relentlessly stay the same?

Track, notice, and keep asking yourself... *"And then what happens?"*

*Somatic Experiencing* takes a hopeful perspective to trauma that aligns with my beliefs. It asserts that our bodies and minds are innately designed to heal from even the most intense experiences and that the effects of trauma are *not* a life-sentence. This approach promotes resiliency and the capacity to heal. It can help us to gently integrate difficult life experiences and increase capacity, energy, and goodness in our lives.

**Survival Energy**

*Somatic Experiencing* is interested in the nervous system's natural defensive responses of animals. There is a threat response cycle that is activated when something in the environment triggers it, and it goes in this order:

- Startle Response:
  - Orienting/looking around to sense if there is a real threat
- Defensive Responses (life or death energy):
  - Fight or Flight: Mobilizing and primitive defensive behaviors are called "fight or flight". If the threat calls for aggression, the animal will fight. If it's unlikely to win a fight, the animal will try to flee.
  - Freeze: If it's deemed that neither fight or flight are good options, the animal will use another line of defense. The freeze response.
- Completion of Survival Response:

    - Discharging the survival energy by: shaking, tremoring, exhaling, crying, laughing, releasing heat, yawning.

The body is wise and knows what it needs to do to protect itself when it is under actual threat. There is no hierarchy of which line of defense is "better". The body places no judgment on these responses. The only goal is to survive the situation and then deal with the consequences later.

From this perspective, this is again why it is less about the specific event itself to determine trauma. The focus is on if the threat response cycle gets interrupted before the completion stage can fully discharge the survival energy.

So, even after we survive an overwhelming experience, our system can remain stuck in one of the defensive responses (fight/flight/freeze). SE is a way of working with this leftover survival energy, allowing the body to process and discharge any leftover energy that may be keeping a person stuck.

### Discharging Survival Energy

SE focuses a lot on discharging survival energy that has been stuck in the nervous system. Discharge can show up as:

- Shaking or trembling
- Heat, warmth, sweating
- Tingling or vibration
- Spontaneous exhale
- Muscular release in some part of the body
- Burping or gurgling in the belly
- Laughing or crying or another emotional release

There are many other frameworks, modalities, and cultures who understand the benefits of discharging survival energy. **This truly is ancient wisdom rediscovered many times over.** The culture you were raised in or a somatic technique you were trained in might have similar ways of exploring this concept. I'm attributing credit to where I first heard ideas, but it's unlikely that this is who discovered it first. I strongly encourage you to follow your own curiosities and rabbit holes to learn more, if this sparks interest.

One modality that was personally helpful for me was *Tension & Trauma Releasing Exercises* (*or TRE®*) by *David Berceli*. His modality focuses primarily on intentionally activating the tremor response in our body to shake out the survival energy.

Here are a few key takeaways about this from his book: *The Revolutionary Trauma Release Process*.

- Shaking signals to our brain that we are safe and have survived the threat.
- We've been socialized out of shaking/tremoring. Our primitive body wants to shake, but our mind (and *Life-Scripts*) tell us not to.
- Keeping the energy stuck in our body creates chronic tension patterns.
- When the survival energy is stuck, our nervous system doesn't realize we've survived so it stays in the energy of "life or death"
- For mammals, the freeze response is dangerous until it is discharged. It lowers resiliency and capacity to deal with future threats.

## Building Capacity

Here are two common questions I got from clients during first sessions - along with my frustrating, but accurate responses:

> Client: "How do we do trauma work in therapy?"
>
> Me: "We go slow. And we get curious."
>
> Client: 🤔
>
> Client: "How long will it take?"
>
> Me: "It takes as long as it takes. The fastest way to heal... is slowly"
>
> Client: 😨

Now, I didn't leave people hanging with *only* those unsatisfying answers. But I did want to start there and set expectations. Working with trauma in a nervous system informed way is different from what many people expect. We don't go straight to the core of the hardest and worst part. We work on the periphery.

Slowly.

Gradually over time the straitjacket of trauma becomes undone.

This approach promotes working with little bits of content at a time. We work on the outer edges of the trauma. Small bits at a time to not overwhelm or re-traumatize. Each little bit builds on each other. Slowing down, in this type of work, is important because the body and the instinctive parts of the brain take longer to process information than the cognitive parts of the brain. We can't just think our way out of trauma. We need to meet the body and nervous system where they are.

There are two important concepts to explore when it comes to building capacity in the nervous system:

**Titration and Pendulation**

Remember... titration = little bits at a time.

If the beaker example explaining titration from the psychedelic dosing chapter didn't resonate. Maybe try this metaphor. I heard it from *Anne Lamott* in *Bird by Bird,* but she was quoting *E.L. Doctorow.*

> *"Writing a novel is like driving a car at night. You can see only as far as your headlights, but you can make the whole trip that way. You don't have to see where you're going, you don't have to see your destination or everything you will pass along the way. You just have to see two or three feet ahead of you."*

If neither beaker nor driving metaphors work for you, ask your favorite search engine this question:

***"How do you eat an elephant?"***

---

Next up: Pendulation

For this explanation, I invite you to bring to mind an image of a pendulum.

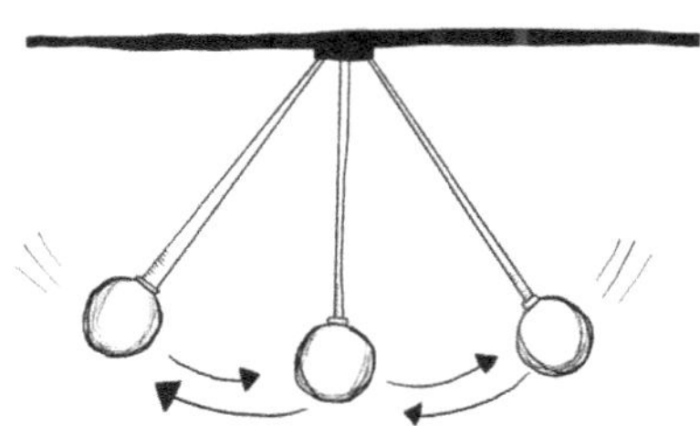

The back and forth movement is essential here. Our nervous systems have the innate capacity to flow back and forth between contraction and expansion. It's the natural rhythm and a sign of a healthy nervous system. *Somatic Experiencing* depicts this through two vortexes.

The **Trauma Vortex** and the **Counter Vortex**.

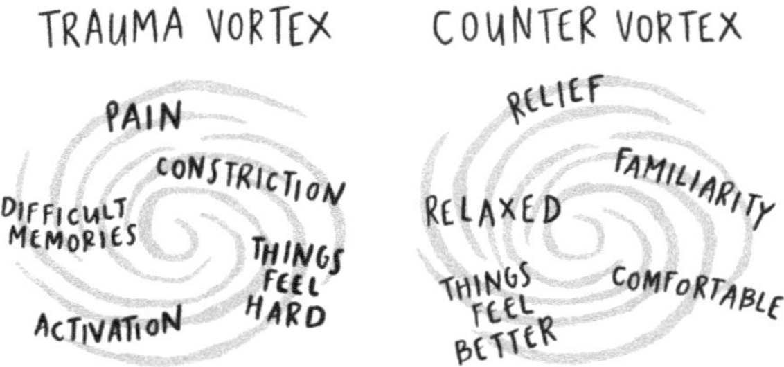


Healing (and accessing more regulation in the nervous system) doesn't come from setting up camp in either one of these vortexes. It's not achieved by going directly to the trauma to "deal with it".

But, it also doesn't happen by bypassing the work, going to the counter vortex and pretending *"Everything is fine!"*

Instead, the healing comes when you're able to pendulate between the two vortexes.

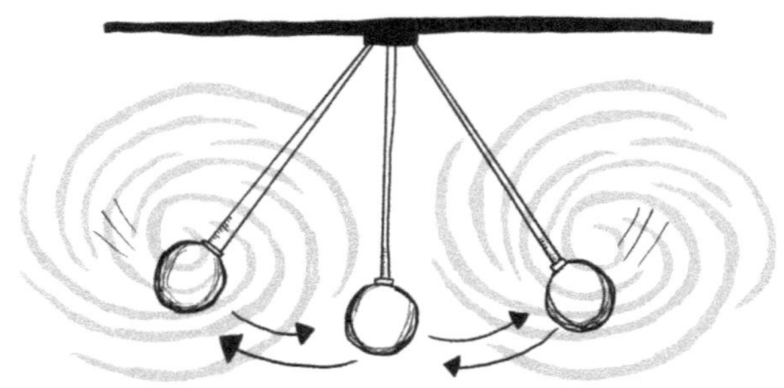

One way to think about this is when you're moving back and forth between the trauma vortex and the counter vortex, the stuck survival energy (fight/flight/freeze) gets "unlocked" and you can begin to discharge it from your body.

**Discharging survival energy = healing the trauma stored in your body**

Understanding pendulation and titration on a fundamental level is why I give those annoying answers to people during first sessions when they are desperate to move through the trauma healing process as fast as possible.

The truth isn't always convenient.

As I was consulting my massive notebook from my 3-year training in *Somatic Experiencing* for these chapters, I found a note I'd written to myself about my own healing journey:

> "The more I let go of the timeline around healing, the more space I make for my body's holding patterns to let go on their own. The more I try to force, the more my body clamps and shuts down. By honoring the "No" of my body and the "I need a break", the more my body is going to trust me and learn that it doesnt have to clamp down and protect itself. My body is going to learn it's not all on its own anymore to protect itself."

Surprise, surprise. So much of this comes back to building trust... with myself.

# [ 52 ]
# FAWNING + FITTING IN

In addition to our fight/flight and freeze responses, there are two additional survival responses with growing research.

**"Fawning" and "Fitting in".**

If you're interested to learn more about these responses, especially as a woman, I encourage you to read *Kimberly Ann Johnson's* book, *Call of the Wild: How We Heal Trauma, Awaken Our Power, and Use It For Good.*

I've had a parasocial mentoring relationship with Kimberly for nearly a decade (*she catalyzed my podcast obsession*) and she has a gift for breaking down and then reconnecting all things related to trauma, sex, and the nervous system.

Remember how I said earlier that the Parasympathetic Nervous System (PNS) is pretty complex? Well, there's one more layer of complexity I want to share with you. Specifically how it can apply to you if you've ever considered yourself a "people-pleaser" or had difficulty setting boundaries.

Beyond supporting rest and sense of ease, the ventral vagal part of the PNS also acts as the "social nervous system". Connection is its superpower. This aspect is specific to mammals and it's the part of our nervous system that is responsible for facial expressions and how we interact and communicate with others.

It's also what allows us to bond with others.

When it's under threat, it resorts to either "fawning" or "fitting in" to survive.

**Fawning** is becoming "nicer" and "less threatening" in order to deescalate a threat. This happens when your body perceives it to be safer to stay in close proximity to a threat vs having the threat waiting out in the shadows for you.

**Fitting in** is when you camouflage yourself in order to avoid the risk of standing out.

Our innate desires to belong, which is necessary for survival, can keep us in the harmful relationship dynamics of fawning and fitting in.

Often, the part of you that uses people-pleasing tendencies or "being a chameleon", feels as though these roles are absolutely necessary for survival. When you can understand the intention behind the roles, you can expand your capacity to have compassion and understanding for these parts of yourself. Which, in and of itself, can begin to change things.

This is also why questioning the *Life-Scripts* you've been handed can register as dangerous in the nervous system, because it can threaten your belonging (and therefore, your survival).

**If fawning or fitting in has been a go-to survival skill for you, it makes sense that:**

- Setting boundaries can feel existential.
- Disagreeing can feel existential.
- It's difficult to discern between your "Yes" and your "No".
- Prioritizing others' needs feels safer.

As with all things nervous system related, I want to encourage you to go slowly with all of this. Remember, titration.

You want to *gradually* expand your capacity for difficult conversations. Start first, with people who feel safer to disagree with. And start with less charged topics. You don't have to do all of this at once.

Explore one *Life-Script* at a time.

Start by just getting curious about how a "Yes" feels in your body. And how your body communicates "No". You don't have to do anything with this information yet. Just allow yourself to be curious and learn more about yourself in the process.

Like all of the survival patterns that can get stuck in your nervous system, fitting in and fawning will take time to unwind.

Curiosity > Judgment is critical to sustainable change in our nervous system. Because, in my experience, judgment most often leads to defensiveness. And defensiveness, by design, is the shield against change.

Next up, let's explore how all of this nervous system information fits into *The Self-Trust Compass*...

[ 53 ]

# SOUTH: REGULATION

**How do you learn you can trust someone?**

Your body sends signals of safety.

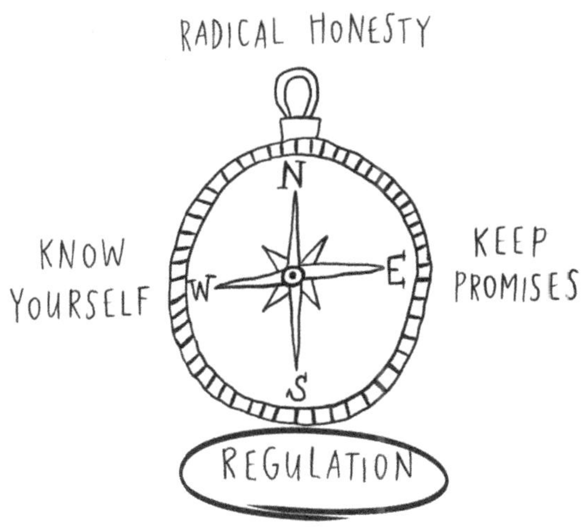

But it's not quite as easy as saying *"Just trust your gut!"* Nervous system regulation is South on the compass - at the base - because it is so foundational to this work of building more trust in yourself.

One job of your nervous system is to scan your environment for possible dangers and alert you if there is a threat. Like when you arrive at the coffee shop for a first date and you go to give an awkward hello hug to the person you've been chatting with for a week, your body recoils and you get a pit in your stomach.

Your body is saying "No!" even if your mind doesn't understand why.

When your nervous system is functioning optimally, it's able to detect possible threats and alert you to respond appropriately to survive. Then - the really important part - once the danger has passed, your system is able to return back to a regulated state of calm. The optimal state of the nervous system is flowing between activation and settling. Contraction and expansion.

The problem that often occurs after prolonged stress or trauma getting stuck in the body, is the nervous system doesn't have capacity to return to a state of regulation. It knows how to activate, but not how to settle. So it gets "stuck on" in a sympathetic arousal or "stuck off" in a parasympathetic state.

**It is really difficult to trust your intuition when your nervous system is dysregulated.**

Like... REALLY hard.

If your nervous system is "stuck on" it might start to see everything and everyone as dangerous. Everything is perceived as a threat. Your system begins to exist only in the activated, anxious, hyper-vigilant state.

*Two problems with this:*

1. **If everything is a threat, nothing is.** Being stuck in danger mode all the time eliminates your ability to discern when a *real* threat is actually present, so you can't protect yourself.
2. **Constant activation is literally exhausting.** Survival mode requires an immense amount of life force energy. Staying there long term exhausts all aspects of your body and can lead to serious health issues.

Relationally, being "stuck on" can show up as someone who builds brick walls with electric fences around themselves to keep people out. This person perceives everyone as potentially dangerous so she won't allow anyone inside.

If your nervous system is "stuck off" you may find yourself numb and disconnected from any red flags in another person, leaving you vulnerable to harm, time and time again.

When you're unable to return to a state of regulation in your nervous system on a regular basis, you lose your discernment superpowers that we spoke about earlier. When you're stuck in survival mode, it's really difficult to connect to the subtitles of your inner voice and wisdom.

There are good reasons you disconnected from your inner voice and intuition. Usually, it starts from a place of protection and survival. And then, you learn to *stay* disconnected. It starts to feel safer to operate from your head and external guidance.

Going inside and reconnecting with your body's wisdom can feel really intimidating and even scary. Especially if you've been disconnected for a long time.

With all of this information, you might see the importance of nervous system regulation, but you might still be wondering...

**"Okay, but how do I ACTUALLY do it?"**

This is a great question and I'm going to give you plenty of ideas to explore on your own. But first, I really want to encourage you to **give yourself the gift of a solid foundation**.

I know it's not always fun and exciting to return to the basics. But the fundamentals are there for a reason. You could go down social media rabbit holes right now and find 50 different nervous system "tricks" and ways to biohack your way to regulation. But, if you bypass the basics, any results you see will likely be temporary.

> **Quickest Way to Biohack Your Nervous System: Do the simple and boring things consistently instead of wasting your time chasing "hacks".**

When you start with the basics and build a solid foundation, you'll be much better able to discern what nervous system advice you want to listen to from others.

Here are the **5 Areas of Regulation** I encourage people to start with:

- **Fuel (food + water)**
- **Movement**
- **Sleep**
- **Sunlight**
- **Connection (nature + others)**

Start by taking a *radically honest* look at what you're currently doing in each of these areas. Get clarity about your starting point:

- **Fuel**
    - How are you currently fueling your body?
    - What foods are you eating?
    - How much and what kind of water are you drinking?
- **Movement**
    - How are you moving your body?
    - What's your relationship to movement?
    - How are you resting your body?
    - What's your relationship to rest?
- **Sleep**
    - How's your sleep quality right now?
    - How much sleep are you getting regularly?
- **Sunlight**
    - How much sunlight are you getting?
    - When are you getting sunlight?
- **Connection**
    - How connected are you feeling to something outside of you?
    - When was the last time you had a soul-nourishing moment with another person?
    - How often are you getting into nature?

**Questions for all areas:**

- Are you not getting enough in any of these areas?
- Are you getting too much in any of these areas?

Once you know your starting point with regulation, there are a few different ways I typically encourage people to proceed. But they all incorporate some aspect of titration. It's most beneficial if you're able to care for yourself in each of these areas every day. But you don't have to start there.

Instead, start with just one area. Choose one area to focus on for one week. Then, choose one small shift you can make in that area.

**Examples of small shifts:**

- Get 5 minutes of sunlight when you first wake up.
- Hug someone for 10 seconds.
- Find the most nutrient dense foods available to you. Eat one of them.
- Put your feet in the dirt for 10 minutes.
- Disconnect from technology early to support better sleep.
- Take a 30 second dance break... RIGHT NOW... Yes, I'm serious.

Building a strong foundation for nervous system regulation isn't something you can "hack" in just a few days. But, when you combine the principles of *Keep Promises* with *Regulation*, you set yourself up for long-term success.

After you're consistently supporting your nervous system in one area, add another area for a week. Once you're consistent with two, add a third. Until you're able to regularly nurture yourself in each area, every day.

When these **5 Areas of Regulation** become part of your daily habits and you consistently do them over time, you foster a healthy nervous system that is resilient and capable of doing deeper healing work.

---

This approach is not about prescribing to you the "right" way to eat, move your body, or connect to others. It's actually an invitation for you to tune deeper into yourself for those answers. Some days you need more food or more sleep. Other days, the answer is less sunlight or less movement.

Also, if you're currently menstruating, this is an opportunity to tune into how your needs may shift and fluctuate throughout your cycle. Where you're at in your cycle can impact your needs for each of these areas.

As you begin to tend to your body more intentionally and incorporate some of these regulation practices, I encourage you to reflect:

- *How does your body respond when you nurture it more?*
- *How are you impacted emotionally and mentally when you prioritize connecting with and caring for your body?*

In upcoming chapters, I'm going to share more specific regulation practices you can try out. But for now, I want to plant some seeds. I want to share some ideas for ways you can build upon the solid foundation of regulation. Ideas to bring you in deeper connection with your body and with yourself. These practices were baked into daily life for many cultures. They don't even have to think about doing it. But for many of us in the overly stressed modern culture of the West, we have to bring a lot of intention to making these things happen. This is by no means an exhaustive list, but a chance to see what ideas you're drawn to. Notice if you feel a 'Yes' in your body to any of them.

**Advanced Regulation Practice Ideas:**

- Breathwork
- Yoga practices
- Drumming
- Movement techniques
- Cold plunging
- Sauna
- Forest bathing
- Meditation
- Trauma release exercises
- Chanting + singing
- Energy healing

[ 54 ]

# MANTRAS FOR REGULATION:

- I will care for my body, mind, and soul.
- I will connect with my aliveness.
- I will listen to myself to better understand what I need.

[ 55 ]

# DENY, DENY, DENY

*"The emotional pain we carry within us isn't just in our head. It's also etched in our muscles."*
*-David Berceli*

I've seen the "trauma" conversation shift quite a bit over the past decade. In many ways the word has been watered down and has lost some of its meaning because people are now claiming everything is "trauma." But if everything is being labeled as trauma, we lose the ability to articulate the nuance inside the spectrum of painful experiences, feeling hurt, and actual trauma responses. "Trauma" has become a placeholder word for almost anything we didn't like that happened to us and a way to put someone on a pedestal - claiming they are "trauma-informed."

That being said, the majority of the people I saw in my therapy office landed further to the *other side* of this cultural shift.

The people I saw most frequently wanted to deny or minimize the painful experiences from their past. And they usually had very good (and often unconscious) reasons for it.

**But denying your past doesn't make it go away.**

The problem with denying or minimizing your past experiences is that you can't heal from something if you don't acknowledge it first. It's one of the *Radical Honesty* mantras for a reason: "*I can only heal what I first acknowledge.*"

Keeping something in your unconscious - gives it a ton of power.

Minimization and denial of past trauma blocks your ability to trust yourself. Because there is a level of dishonesty at play - even when it's not intentional. There is a part of you that might be trying to protect you by denying or minimizing your past. But the alternate version of reality isn't fully truthful. And remember, even when people have the best intentions for lying to us - we still don't trust them.

This isn't encouraging a life sentence of victimhood. Not at all.

Because here's the thing...

**Whether you're denying that you experienced trauma or you're defining yourself by the trauma you experienced - the *trauma* is still controlling you.**

Sometimes, suffering comes from avoiding your story. And sometimes, suffering comes from clinging to your story. You might experience both sides of this suffering paradox in your healing journey...

Maybe you first face the difficult truth - that you've been avoiding your pain. You've been minimizing your experiences as a way to not face the reality of their impact. Deeply wishing that the things that happened to you - *didn't*. Maybe you even try some bypassing routes to survive in the world.

Makes sense.

And then at some point, maybe you begin down the path of acknowledging reality. You stop denying. You step out of wishful thinking and accept what happened. And then - maybe you start to cling to the story. What happened *to* you - starts to define you. You try on victim labels and they feel important because you're finally honoring the parts of you that were harmed.

Again. Makes sense.

But I'm going to assert that *neither* of these expected waypoints are where you want your final destination to be.

Because neither gives you an internal locus of control.

You'll need different things along the way. The antidote when you're stuck in an avoidance cycle will be different than when you're clinging to the story of what happened to you.

But the thing that's really helpful regardless of where you are along the journey is something we've already talked about.

*Radical Honesty.*

Acknowledging painful moments from your past allows you to be honest about your starting point. It can be an empowering experience. Once you accept the reality of what happened in your life, you get to take an active role in your own healing.

*To be very clear* - "accepting the reality" that something happened is *not* condoning the behavior or abuse.

**But what happened *to* you does not have to define you.**

One way to explore your past experiences is to make a *Both/And List.* This is a way to acknowledge multiple truths at the same time.

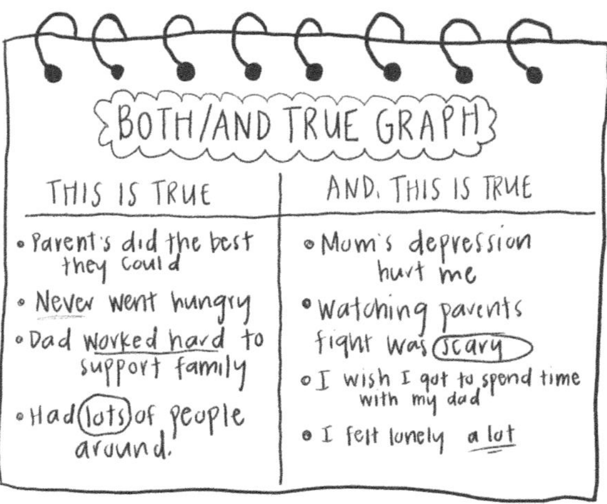


Another example of how denial and minimization can impact your trust in yourself is by misattributing your pain or stress. We talked about this in the *Radical Honesty* chapter and it also fits in with the *Regulation* practices you're beginning to implement.

Bringing more regulation into your nervous system doesn't automatically fix everything. **All the morning sunlight in the world isn't going to change a fundamental misalignment in your marriage**. But focusing on those basics *can* expand your capacity to tune into your body and listen for what's really out of alignment in your life.

# [ 56 ]
# GUIDED SOMATIC PRACTICES

Here are some of my favorite somatic practices that you can use to build on the solid foundation of nervous system *Regulation* you've established:

- **Somatic Opposites**
  - When you're ready to build up your discernment muscles even more.
- **SE Resourcing**
  - Orienting, Self-Contact, Grounding
- **5 Senses with Tea**
  - Get into the present moment.

- **Resourcing with 5 Senses**
    - SOS - feel better soon.
- **Longer Exhale**
    - When you're struggling with anxiety.
- **Energy [mine + not mine]**
    - For all the empaths out there...
- **Cranial-Occipital Hold**
    - A technique in craniosacral therapy where one hand gently cradles the occiput (back of the skull) while the other rests on the frontal bone. It's a hold you can also do for yourself.
        - Once you have your hands in place, play around with the amount of pressure you want to apply.
        - Once you find the right amount of pressure, hold for several minutes inviting your exhale to lengthen.

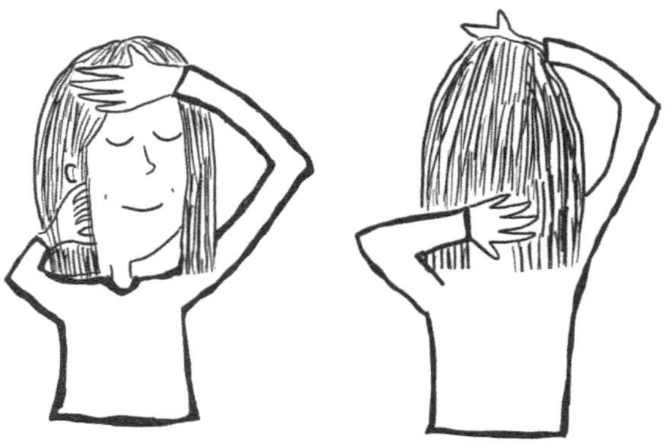

# [ 57 ]
# CONVERGENCE

Remember, The *Self-Trust Model*™ exists at the convergence of somatic therapy, "parts work", and psychedelic therapy (with or without medicine).

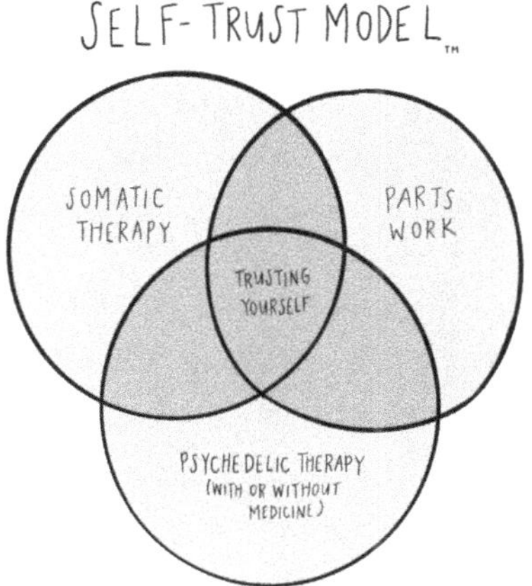


All throughout this book, I've been alluding to the "parts" in me. Sometimes, I've even been presumptuous about your parts. I apologize if I've been wildly misguided and you, in fact, are a fully one dimensional creature and can't relate to any of this "parts talk." Though, I'm guessing if you were that offended, you wouldn't have stuck around long enough to be reading this section of the book.

But for those of you who weren't offended by my presumption, *"Hey!"*

> *"Hey!"* - to the part of you who deeply resonates with the idea of having many (sometimes conflicting) parts inside.
>
> *"Hey!"* - to the part who is a little worried that acknowledging all your parts might mean you need to do a brain scan. (It *probably* doesn't.)

There's a reason I didn't start this book with definitions about the parts model I was trained in, *Internal Family Systems,* and explaining what I mean when I say "parts of you", even though I think definitions are helpful.

What I've seen in my work with people is we often don't need this explained. It's an innate knowing, deep inside us. The complicated nature of our psyche makes sense because we live it every day. The *IFS* framework just puts language to what our soul already knows.

There is power in putting words to our experiences, for sure, which is why I'm offering that to you now. And, if I'm being really honest, I've got intellectual parts of me that *love* understanding how things fit together as part of the bigger picture. These are the parts that use logic and graphs to help me "buy into" what my body already knows.

So, I'm still going to give you an overview of the *IFS* framework. Just in case you have parts who want that too.

# [ 58 ]
# INTERNAL FAMILY SYSTEMS® OVERVIEW

The *Internal Family Systems* (*IFS*) framework asserts that the human mind is subdivided into a number of different "parts" or sub-personalities. The belief is that we have an entire family of parts inside each of us. Therefore, family systems theories can be applied to the internal system in each one of us.

One of my favorite aspects of the *IFS* approach is that it takes a non-pathologizing view of the human experience. We don't need to slap a diagnosis onto everyone. There are no "bad" parts. And we're not broken for having a multitude of parts inside us.

In addition to an abundance of parts, everyone also has a Self (with a capital S).

Self can, and optimally should, be the leader of the internal system. You can think of this as having Self-leadership.

**How do you know what is Self and what is a part of you?**

Capital S - Self - has 8 qualities to look out for. And thankfully, for all our alliteration-loving parts, the founder of *IFS*, Dr. Richard Schwartz, was able to find a way to make them all start with the letter C.

**8 C's of Self Energy:**

- Compassion
- Creativity
- Curiosity
- Confidence
- Courage
- Calmness
- Connectedness
- Clarity

In addition to Self existing in all of us, it's also true that Self is always present. Even when we can't see it or feel it, it's always there.

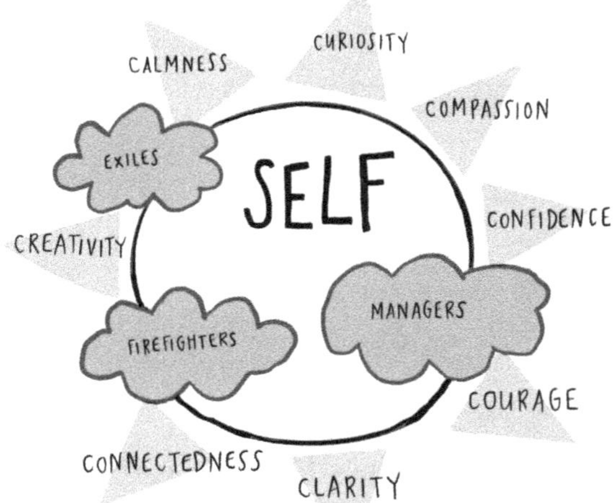

You can think of Self as the sun. Even when the clouds have fully covered the sun and you can't see the bright rays or feel the warmth, it's there. Even when day has turned to night and the dawn of the morning feels lightyears away, the sun still exists. Even during the seasons of life that feel like you're barely surviving an Alaskan winter, the sun is relentless.

The 8 qualities of Self energy help us to know when the sun is shining brightly. But being Self-led in our life is not about being fully "in" Self energy or "out" of Self energy. It's not all or nothing. It's a spectrum. You can begin to ask yourself:

**How much Self energy do I have access to right now, in this moment?**

The reason it's important to access as much Self energy as possible is because this is where our innate healing wisdom resides. When we're able to make decisions and communicate with others from as much Self energy as possible, life is more peaceful, we have better relationships, and we're connected to our integrity.

However, our parts can get in the way of this. They are the clouds (*or the Alaskan winter*). They can act in some pretty extreme and destructive ways at times.

At the core, **IFS is a loving way of relating internally to all your parts and externally to the people in your life.** Let's first explore the relationship between Self and your parts.

IFS breaks down our "parts" into three categories:

- Exiles
- Managers
- Firefighters

WE ALL HAVE MULTIPLE PARTS
(SUB-PERSONALITIES)
PROTECTOR PARTS
EXILES
(WOUNDED PARTS)
PARTS THAT HAVE BEEN WOUNDED + HURT
CAN GET FROZEN AT AGE THEY WERE WOUNDED.
MANAGERS
(PREVENTATIVE PARTS)
THEY TRY TO PREVENT THE WOUNDS FROM BEING TRIGGERED
EXAMPLES: INNER CRITIC
PEOPLE PLEASING
PERFECTIONISM
NEEDING TO BE LIKED
FIREFIGHTERS
(REACTIVE PARTS)
THEY REACT ONCE WOUND IS TRIGGERED.
ONE JOB: STOP THE PAIN
EXAMPLES: NUMBING OUT
SUBSTANCE USE
SHOPPING
BINGING
ALL PARTS HAVE POSITIVE INTENT. EVEN THE MOST DESTRUCTIVE ONES

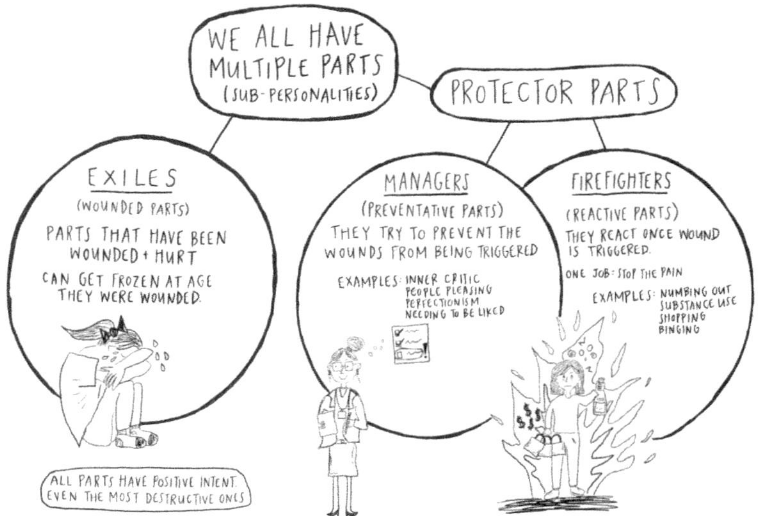

## Exiles

- These are our wounded parts that carry the burdens of past pain we've experienced. They carry the stories and narratives of: "I'm bad", "I'm broken", "I'm not good enough", and "I'm not worthy".
- They can get "stuck" at the age they were wounded. Think: "my little 5 year old inside" or the teenager part that gets activated every time you see a group of middle school girls laughing. *Oh, that one's just me?*
- These wounds are carried subconsciously and in your nervous system. They are often very painful to look at so we push them into the dark corners of our psyche.

Before we connect with our exiles, we want to first get permission from their protectors. We have two types of protector parts, and we'll talk about both. But it's important to remember that all of them take on their roles to try and keep us safe. They all have positive and benevolent intentions.

## Managers

- You can think of them as *preventative* protectors. They try to prevent old wounds (exiles) from being triggered.
- Their motto: "NEVER AGAIN!"
    - Whatever the experience was that caused the wounding, the managers are here to say "Never again!" They will do anything it takes to make sure that specific pain never happens again.
- Many of these Managers are praised and reinforced by our society.
    - "Look how organized you are!", "Thank you for being so helpful all the time!", "You're so easy to get along with!", "I love how independent you are!"

## Firefighters

- You can think of them as the *reactive* protectors. They react once the wound (exile) has been triggered.
- Their motto: "STOP THE PAIN IMMEDIATELY!"
    - Their only job is to stop the pain - at any and all costs. Firefighters do not care about damaging your leather couch or pricy artwork with the water they are using to put out the fire.
- Firefighters are often looked down on, by society and by our Managers.
    - "They're just trying to get attention.", "Why can't they just stop drinking?", "She just needs to eat a cheeseburger.", "Geez, why are you so forgetful."

This might be a nice time to remind you that all protector parts have positive intentions, even the most destructive ones. Even the ones you hate most in yourself. It doesn't mean their impact in your life has been good, but their intentions are always benevolent.

The goal of IFS work is not to eliminate any of these parts, but instead to help them find more beneficial roles within the system. We want to differentiate Self from these parts and empower Self to be the effective leader of the family. This way, all the parts can have a voice. They can all have a seat at the table in the boardroom and have their opinions heard. But ultimately...

**Self is the one who makes the final decision.**

When our protector parts are able to feel the presence of Self, they begin to feel safe to step out of their protective roles. The tunnel vision they've had begins to widen and they can see they aren't all alone to fix the problem anymore. The entire system can settle and find more peace.

This can be described as building the "Self-to-part" relationship. At the very core - **this is *relational work.*** It's about building trust between Self and all the exiles, managers, and firefighters. In the upcoming chapters, we'll get practical with exercises to support this relationship and how this perspective can foster more Self-Trust.

---

As I shared earlier in this chapter, this framework is also about lovingly relating to the external relationships in your life. Imagine for a moment that you have space to choose who is going to react when your husband once again forgets to plan date night when it's his turn, even after you reminded him yesterday.

*Who do you want to respond?*

- Your 5 year old little girl with abandonment wounds?
- Your overly controlling manager?
- Your "get on the first flight out of town" firefighter?

*Or do you want Self to respond?*

---

**Practices to connect with more Self energy:**

- 8 C's of Self Meditation Guided Meditation

- Choose one of the 8 C's of Self to focus on for a week. *We'll go with "Courage" for this example.* Each time you find yourself stuck at a decision-making crossroads, ask yourself:

*What is the most courageous option I could choose?*

# [ 59 ]

# HEAD EAST AGAIN...

Now that you have the IFS language to understand "parts", I encourage you to return to the *Keep Promises* chapter. Revisit the idea of setting commitments from Self energy. I'll even make it easy on you... **it's on page 212**.

*With this new perspective, how does the concept of keeping the "right" promises land for you now?*

This is a reminder that these directions are not linear. And it's not a checklist. It's expected that you will revisit all the directions many times over. As you gain a new awareness or perspective, you can revisit a direction or chapter and see how you want to approach it with the new information.

[ 60 ]

# TWO FACED FEAR

F*ear* has come to tea many times by now. She has a standing Thursday at 4pm tea time appointment and yet, she's still the first to snag an extra opening in my schedule.

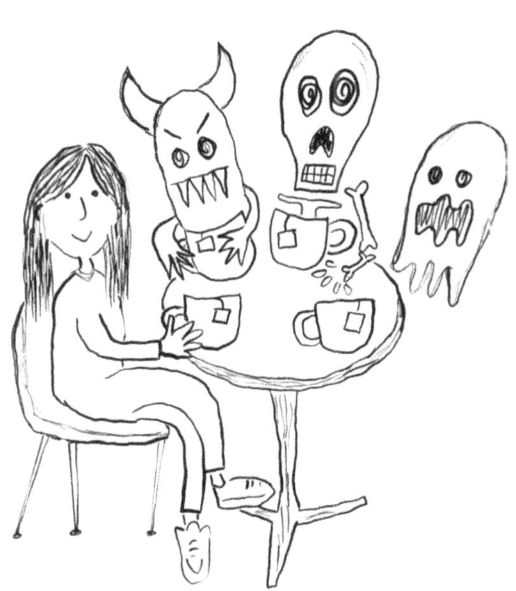

Mostly, *Fea*r tells me how much better other people are at the things I want to do. She shares all the elaborate stories of how things won't work out, and how I'll end up broke and alone.

Recently though, something *else* slipped into the same long monologue I'd heard a hundred times about how I'm not "good enough". It was barely noticeable at first and *Fear* continued rambling so fast I almost missed it. But with a little redirection, she said it again.

I sat there, stunned. Unable to continue enjoying the matcha in front of me.

*Did she really say that?*

Fuck, it's even more cliché than I could've scripted.

She's not really afraid of being bad at writing.

She's afraid she might be good enough that people will actually want to read it.

## [ 61 ]
## FAILURE

The obvious direction for my business to go after I closed my therapy practice was group work. I'd been offering retreats for over a year at this point. They were bringing in good income for my business. I had a waitlist of 20+ women for the next round of *Adventure Club*. The third season *should* have been easier to fill than the first two. Everyone who had completed the first two seasons wanted more. They'd all been telling me how much they wanted an alumni retreat. Doubling down on more groups and retreats made logical sense.

I found myself thinking... *"I can't wait to run this next season, it should be so much easier this time!"*

> *Are the words "logical" and "should" enough foreshadowing by now?*

Turns out, it *wasn't* as easy as I thought it should be.

And maybe, that's because I made a fundamental change to the structure of *Adventure Club*, **for all the wrong reasons**.

Part of what makes *Adventure Club* so special is that we move at the *"Speed of Trust"*. Not logical trust, but the embodied *experience* of trust. It was very intentionally set up in a way for trust with the other members to build organically over time.

That's why having multiple retreats is a crucial component. This set-up removes the pressure of only meeting for a single retreat - often resulting in forced vulnerability amongst the members. The multi-retreat structure was meant to allow trust and connection to deepen each time we came back together. With plenty of space for integration in between retreats.

I took something that makes *Adventure Club* so transformational - and chucked it right out the window. All because I was feeling the pressure to monetize quickly. To scale my business. To prove something. I tried turning *Adventure Club* into any other genetic week-long retreat with personal growth ideas, movement practices, and sharing circles.

But I wasn't ready to take responsibility for this error in judgment right away. Instead, I was briefly tempted by the "woe is me" narrative. I was almost fully pulled under by the riptide of unnecessary suffering. The kind of suffering that comes when we think we're entitled to life the way we think it *should* be.

I sat with myself on the day I *should* have been celebrating the next season of "Adventure Sisters". The day I had planned to offer gratitude and energetically welcome them into the community of the seasons before.

So why instead, am I sitting at my computer looking at a combined total of exactly...

**ZERO signups**?

*Doubt* filled the silence with some rapid fire answers:

*Doubt: "Because you're a terrible retreat leader and no one likes you!"*

*Doubt: "Because The Self-Trust Model is stupid and no one cares!"*

*Doubt: "Because all that 'transformation' you witnessed was just a fluke!"*

*Doubt: "Because it was a terribly reckless idea to close your therapy practice and now the universe is punishing you!"*

Okay, wow. I have to stop you there, *Doubt*. Don't you think that last one is getting a little egotistical? Do you really think the universe cares *that* much about your little retreats?

**Any other parts have something they want to get off their chest?**

Per usual, *Fear* doesn't need to wait for her standing tea time appointment with me. She jumps right in:

*Fear: "You know you're going to lose everything, right?"*

*Fear: "I hope you still remember how to smile and nod at strangers' stupid jokes about your height, because you're going to be back waiting tables again very soon."*

*Fear: "You seriously think you can have a baby now? With no income?"*

It takes everything I have in me not to break down after the final jab from *Fear*. She knows just how to cut me. All she's ever had to do my whole life is plant the seed that I don't care about someone else. She just has to allude that my decision is selfish in some way, and I immediately turn my power over to her.

But it's not quite that simple anymore.

Just because she knows how to scare me, doesn't mean she gets to make my decisions.

I take a few breaths in a paper bag while everyone else gets a chance to speak up. Once all my parts feel seen and heard, my body settles a bit.

Then, a quiet and steady voice meets my eardrums. It takes me a second to recognize that the sounds I'm hearing are coming from my own vocal cords. It's disorienting in the same way as hearing your voice on a recording.

The voice, *my voice*, says:

> **"I can't wait to see what happens in October instead."**

The sentiment of the words sink in. I feel my Self energy expand throughout my entire body. I feel calm and steady. I feel clarity in my body, even though it's not logical clarity yet. It feels like the universe is winking at me. Things make sense (*even though they don't really make sense at all*). I actively feel myself detaching from any particular outcome.

I'm rattled away from my center once again when even more parts begin to chime in:

> *The Optimist: "There's probably something really awesome that's going to happen in the fall instead of running these groups! I can't wait to see what it is!"*
>
> *Doubt: "Well that's a hope strategy if I've ever seen one!"*
>
> *The Writer: "This is going to make a great chapter in a book one day..."*

Before *Fear* can jump in with another gut punch, I exhaustedly interject:

*"Great, thank you all for showing up today. But maybe next time, this could just be an email?"*

[ 62 ]

# WEST: KNOW YOURSELF

**How do you learn you can trust someone?**

You get to know them and overtime you learn if you can trust them or not.

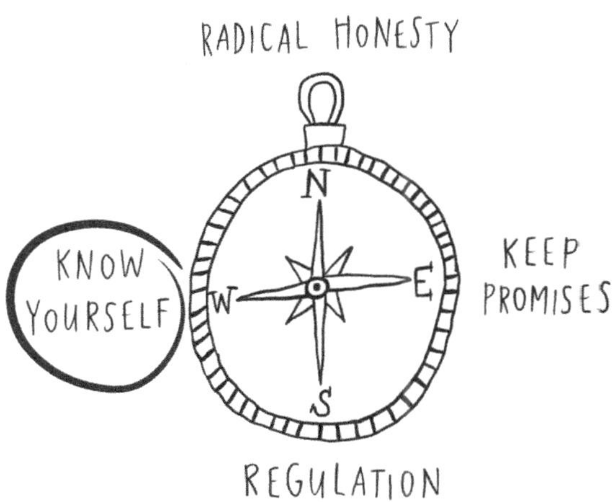

When you first meet someone, it's healthy to have a neutral level of trust. It's not necessarily beneficial to assume the worst in everyone you meet, but a stranger has done nothing yet to prove that they're trustworthy to you. So it makes sense that you don't automatically trust them.

Trust is built over time as you get to know someone more and more. And the same applies to trust with yourself.

**Self-awareness is a prerequisite to Self-Trust**.

So if you want to trust yourself more, you've got to stop being a stranger to yourself.

It's just like the marketing adage suggests, we do business with people that we *"Know, Like, and Trust."* It's the same for trusting ourselves. You have to know yourself, before you can like yourself, before you can trust yourself.

I strongly encourage you to slow down and get curious about yourself.

Because the relationship you have with yourself is as important as any other relationship in your life. Actually, I'll put a vote in for the assertion that it's the *most* important relationship you'll ever have. It's the foundation that all other relationships are built on.

*Martha Beck* put it bluntly in her book, *The Way of Integrity*:

> *"Being split from ourselves is hell."*

**What do you imagine life could be like if you took the time to connect and nurture the relationship with yourself the same way you would any other important relationship?**

Well often, getting to know someone involves time.

Quality time together.

You guessed it. The same is true for getting to *Know Yourself.*

## Start With Subtraction

Before we explore ideas of what to **add** to your life as a way to *Know Yourself* better, let's start by exploring what happens when you first **subtract** things from your life.

A key piece of this is decreasing the external noise. Because when the external input is greater than the internal, it's really hard to hear your intuition.

Often, before you can really hear the whisper inside, you must first quiet the external. Disconnect from social media. Turn off the podcasts and news. Actually, maybe go ahead and shut off anything connected to technology.

This is actually a great time to remind you of the "Nature Clarity" we spoke about earlier. Take some time, alone in nature, and allow yourself to get quiet and still.

## What emerges from within?

You might learn more about yourself than just what *Life-Scripts* you're operating from.

Another thing to consider subtracting is any mind-altering substances.

While choosing not to drink alcohol is a decision I made years ago that continues to have long-lasting benefits in my life, I'm not suggesting everyone has to be sober to trust themselves.

But I am saying that constantly relying on alcohol, drugs, and other substances to distract yourself or change your emotional state - can prevent you from knowing yourself as deeply as you may desire.

**Back to Addition**

Here's another idea to get to *Know Yourself* better (so you can trust yourself more).

Imagine you're meeting with a new friend, or going on a first date, or maybe you're nothing like me and you're actually excited about a business networking opportunity.

Choose whichever scenario gets you excited to get to know someone. What questions do you want to ask them?

Now... you probably know where this is going...

Ask yourself those same questions.

**Fake Bonus Points Alert:** Take yourself on a date to *Know Yourself* better.

If you want some ideas on what to do on a solo date, I got you covered.

Now, this is where it gets really "fun".

After you try to sit under a tree in silence for a couple hours, or block social media from your phone, or you try to take yourself out on a date... notice any resistance that arises. Do you have any parts that *don't* want to do this?

- *What are you afraid might happen if you truly knew yourself?*
- *What are your go-to strategies to distract you from knowing yourself?*

For now, just notice it. Try not to push it away. Just allow it to be there. As always, you can offer it some tea. See if these resistant parts have anything more they want to share with you. The first step in knowing yourself more fully is just noticing what happens when you slow down and spend time with yourself.

---

As I've drilled into you enough throughout this book, we're all multidimensional beings. There are many realms you can get to *Know Yourself* better. And exploring any aspect of your life can create a ripple effect in trusting yourself more too.

**Realms to *Know Yourself* Better:**

- Physical
- Mental
- Emotional
- Spiritual
- Financial
- Sexual
- Other areas?

This isn't all or nothing – you might have a really sophisticated understanding of your finances and even why you have the relationship to money that you do, but still have no idea what you want done to you in the bedroom.

Let's bring in some *Radical Honesty* again:

- *Which realms do you already know yourself pretty well?*
- *Which realms are you a stranger to yourself?*
- *Which realms do you desire more connection to yourself?*

One thing I love about this framework is that pretty much ANYTHING can be a portal to *Know Yourself* better (so you can trust yourself more).

Here is a (very incomplete) list of portals to *Know Yourself* better:

- Solo Travel
- Yoga
- Weightlifting
- Cycle Syncing
- Values Exploration (*more to come in the "Winter"*)
- Entrepreneurship
- Hiking/Camping
- Tarot/Oracle Cards (*more to come in the "Winter*)
- Human Design
- Gardening
- Pole Dancing
- Conscious Parenting
- Writing
- Knitting
- Self-Photography
- Personality Tests

Have you explored any of these portals? What did you learn about yourself? What other portals can you think of that you've gotten to know yourself better through?

One final portal I want to share with you now connects back into IFS. It's a way to get to know your parts better and also how they interact with each other.

### Parts Map

You can do this on any kind of paper and use whatever writing utensils you want. Pens, markers, watercolors, crayons, anything. The idea is to create a visual representation of all your parts. Or at least the ones that want to be shown right now. You can use images or words to represent them on the page.

Create it however you'd like. Place each part on the map wherever it wants to be, using whatever medium it wants.

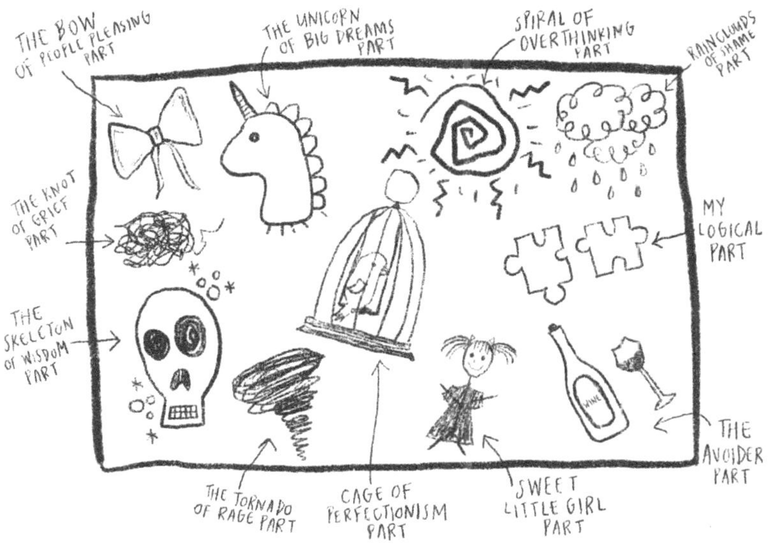

After you're finished, you can return to your map and just notice.

**Notice:**

- Which parts are next to each other?
- Did you choose different mediums for different parts?
- What do you notice about the size of the parts?
- What do you notice in your body when you look at the different parts on your map?

---

Knowing yourself can be a lifelong process if you allow it to be. If you're anything like me, you'll have many evolutions of who you are. Shifting identities. Bardos and liminal in-between spaces to explore. Especially if you give yourself permission in life to change your mind.

That's another reason why you don't have to do all of this immediately. Maybe exploring your sexuality feels really intimidating right now. That's okay. Allow yourself to follow your *current* curiosities. Explore where your soul nudges want to take you in this season of life. Get to know yourself there, first.

These practices will always be here. You, in five years, might have very different ideas about what you want to explore.

Take your time.

All of this - takes as long as it takes.

And hey, maybe you can even let yourself have some fun along the way.

[ 63 ]

## MANTRAS FOR KNOW YOURSELF:

- I will reconnect with myself by spending time alone.
- I will no longer treat myself like a stranger.
- I will find quiet places to listen to myself.

# [ PART 3 ]
# FALL

We celebrate... with the energy of the **Fall Equinox.**

A balance between light and dark.

A time to reap the rewards of the Summer's work.

A time for gratitude.

A time for appreciation.

A metaphorical reminder from the falling leaves to appreciate how beautiful it can be to let go.

A harvesting of the fruits of your labor.

A time to transcend limitations.

The deeper layers of the work begin to reveal themselves...

The parts you couldn't see in the Spring...

Capacity is expanded...

. . .

And we begin to connect the dots.

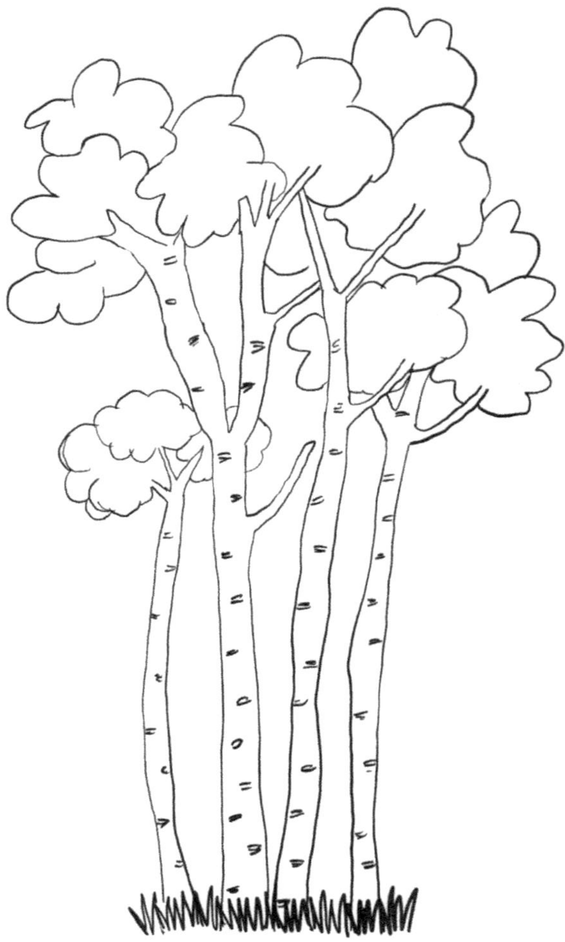

## [ 64 ]

## CONTROLLED BURN

September 22nd

Well... it happened. I wasn't sure if I was going to be able to - but I did.

I burned it all down...

The online group I was running finished last month and just a few days ago, I ran the final monthly meet-up for the Alumni Group. Some were disappointed by the ending. And that makes sense. This pivot didn't just impact me - it impacted them as well.

Even with over a decade of inner work, I still don't like disappointing other people. Especially people I like and love. But I reminded myself what I used to tell my clients:

"Sometimes, you have to disappoint other people to build trust with yourself. It might scare the shit out of your People-Pleaser, but you can still do it."

Just another moment in a long string of similar moments this year. Trusting what I know is right - even when it's hard. And even when I don't fully get it yet.

I let myself be blindsided this summer with a complete re-direction of my business.

I followed through on the commitment to shut down all the groups. (I do hope it came across as the "controlled burn" I intended...)

And I followed through on focusing on only one thing in my business for an entire season.

Today marks the end of that commitment.

And I'm grateful I get to celebrate in my favorite forested city.

This view is one I'll never grow tired of. I'll forever be grateful for all this city, and especially these trees, have given me.

I'm not able to fully connect all the dots about why things needed to unravel the way they did, but I do know one thing with certainty.

If I'd continued to try and do "all the things" - there's no way I'd be publishing my first book next month.

[ 65 ]

# DATING AROUND

Remember the three month commitment I made to myself to focus on only *one* project in my business?

To be exclusive. Monogamous. To go steady with "The 13 Lessons".

Well, to be honest, I doubted if I'd be able to follow through on this one.

And it wasn't surprising to me that it took extreme discipline at times. I was courted by so many other ideas. Other experiences I wanted to create in my business kept checking me out. More than once I even caught *myself* with a wandering eye. And sometimes, I allowed natural flirtation to take over.

I'd recover and quickly say, *"You sound great and all, but I'm not really seeing other ideas right now. Can I circle back to you in, say, September?"*

Maybe these ideas thought I was playing hard to get. But I wasn't.

I *wanted* to scream *"Yes, let's do it!"* to so many of these ideas and begin planning our future together. Especially the tall, dark, and handsome idea of hosting a cozy intention setting weekend retreat in the snow capped mountains of Colorado.

*So much tea... So many cozy sweaters... So much hygge... ahhhh.*

Okay, back to discipline, that's what we're talking about.

Being disciplined is hard. Sometimes, it's *really* hard.

But I'm also reminded that when you make commitments to yourself from a place of Self energy, the "hard" of being disciplined - is the hard I want to choose. These are the "right" promises to keep.

And, if I'm truly meant to create a training program for *The Self-Trust Model*, the idea will still be there next year.

It was another reminder for me to trust my intuition *before* it makes logical sense. And to make space for the "13 Lessons" to evolve into what it was meant to be. Which, as it turns out, is a book.

Not only do I have to get comfortable with calling myself a writer. I also have to play around with the idea of being an author.

When I got the intuitive hit to close my therapy practice, I had no idea that's where it would all lead. I didn't have the complete picture. All I knew is I was setting commitments from Self energy. I knew these were the promises worth keeping. I knew if I wanted to collapse time; a one track mind and consistent follow through would be required.

I knew I couldn't get distracted by shiny objects or an idea with a glistening six-pack.

## [ 66 ]

# REAP THE REWARDS

If I'm being honest, one of the hardest lessons I've repeatedly relearned in my life is how to go *towards* difficult conversations. It's even one of "The 13 Lessons".

*"Lesson #9: Be the Buffalo"* speaks directly to the benefits of facing challenging conversations with the people you love the most. It's this particular lesson that continues to annoy all my avoidant parts. *And yes, there are many.*

But surprisingly, I found that applying this lesson actually creates *more* intimacy in my relationships. On the other side of uncomfortable conversations with people in my life, I actually found a *deeper* connection to them. *Or they ran the other way screaming "Ahhh nooo, not for me!!"* Either way, there's been clarity.

Most often, I found that deeply rooted trust was actually formed *during* the discomfort of real and honest conversations. The conversations where we both value delivering the truth - with kindness. The challenging times strengthened our bond.

Has this ever happened to you? Have you ever felt closer to someone after coming out the other side of the hard conversations trenches with them?

> **What if the same rewards for hard conversations *(connection, intimacy, understanding)* applied to the relationship you have with your inner parts?**

I've found that this perspective helps me "buy-in" to the idea of sitting with my fears, my shame, my doubt, my insecurities, and my pain. I'm not sitting with my feelings just for the sake of it. There is a purpose.

This process creates the foundation for trust to flourish.

# [ 67 ]
# GRATITUDE

In the month leading up to publishing my first book, I focused on three things to help prepare me for "launch day":

1. **Connecting with my hype people.** The ones who don't think I'm crazy for doing this. The ones who cheer me on even more when I want to let *Doubt* or *Fear* make my decisions.
2. **Time in nature.** Lots of long hikes to access "Nature Clarity" and connect me to my "*why*" for doing all of this.
3. **Daily gratitude practice.**

Maybe you read that third one and immediately wanted to respond with...

- *But does a gratitude practice even work?*
- *Isn't the "grateful energy" of the Fall just a construct for spiritual bypassing?*

- *Is it real?*

These are frequent follow up questions whenever I share the idea for someone to try out a gratitude practice. I understand why these questions are so common. They are the same questions I hear when we talk about pulling oracle cards or dream interpretation (*more to come on that*).

Or making a vision board.

Or meeting the needs of your inner child.

Many of us have a part inside who wants to "capital K - Know" that something is real and legit before we spend (*waste?*) time doing it. Maybe we even want to see a peer reviewed journal article to "prove" it. *Although... Does this part care about how a study was conducted to see if it actually applies to them or is it just craving some validation from "science"?*

Regardless, I understand why the question comes up. But I don't have the answer for you. I do, though, have a different question you could ask.

**Is it helpful?**

> Is connecting to your inner child and identifying the needs that weren't met in childhood and then tending to those needs now.... helpful?
>
> Is taking time to yourself in the morning to remember your dreams and understand your subconscious more... helpful?
>
> Is prioritizing time to connect to questions you have inside and then bringing them to an oracle deck and then tapping into what resonates and what doesn't... helpful?

Is slowing down in a chaotic and overstimulated world to connect to things you're grateful for… helpful?

Only you can answer those questions for yourself. And it may take some trial and error, some patience, and some repetition to discover your answers.

I can share my experience with you, though.

My gratitude journaling practice, just like all of my journaling practices, has waxed and waned over the years. And I can always tell what part of this writing lunar cycle I'm in based on how I'm feeling.

It's annoyingly clear and simple. I have a different emotional baseline when I'm consistently practicing gratitude. When I start my mornings by simply writing down three things I'm grateful for, my capacity for the daily turbulence of life is expanded.

So, no. I don't really care about a study from Harvard to tell me if it's "real" or not.

I care about whether it helps me or not.

And in the months leading up to putting my first book into the world, I needed as much help as I could get. *Fear* and *Doubt* were getting LOUD. And when they're constantly trying to get my attention, I get a little cranky. I'm not the most fun person to be around when I'm overthinking and feeling insecure. I didn't want my irritability spilling over into my personal life.

I was publishing a book for the first time and I wanted to enjoy as much of the process as possible. And feel gratitude that it was even a possibility for me. So I made a conscious decision, one month before the publication date, to return to gratitude.

Recognition of three things I was grateful for was the price of entry to begin work each day. And just like every other time in my life I've prioritized this practice, it didn't take long for me to feel the impact.

[ 68 ]

# PERKS OF BEING AN OUTSIDER

S*peaking of gratitude...*

I could fill many chapters with the pitfalls of not knowing anything about the publishing industry. Of not having the necessary connections or even full understanding of when to use a semicolon; *I'm pretty sure I just nailed it, though.*

I could feel sorry for myself and criticize past versions of me for not paying attention in my one English class in college. I could go into a "woe is me" spiral and feel sorry for myself about my starting point.

But honestly, that path isn't even tempting.

Because I know that being an "insider" in any industry comes with a certain level of indoctrination. I experienced it with therapy and I know all too well the level of effort it takes to unlearn everything that was deeply ingrained in me.

---

**Beliefs I *Was* Indoctrinated With as a Therapist:**

- If you share anything about yourself with a client, it will hurt them.
- Preach self-care to your clients, but no, you can't take time off.
- Don't expect to make any money - that's not why you got into this work.
- Your knowledge of specific therapeutic modalities is what will make you a "good therapist".
- If you want to get paid a living wage, you don't actually care about people.
- Don't bring your humanity into the therapy room.
- Boundaries between client and therapist are black and white.
- Show up the same for all of your clients.
- Say this exact thing: "_____" to prove to your clients and colleagues that you're a "good person".

As an outsider to the academic writing and publishing worlds, I've only *heard* from other authors about the beliefs they were indoctrinated with.

**Beliefs I *Wasn't* Indoctrinated With as an Author:**

- Traditional publishing is better than self-publishing.
- You can't make any money being a writer.
- You shouldn't even want to make money writing your books - it's supposed to be about helping people.
- You have to write a book proposal.
- You have to have a literary agent.
- Most books don't sell.
- It takes many many years to get a book published.

- If you get a traditional publishing deal, it means you're a better writer, which means you're a better person. Obviously.

So yeah... I'm really grateful I don't have decades of beliefs to unlearn from the literary world about if it's okay to want to make money and how to be a "good person". It seems everyone has an opinion about that, but I think the therapy world gave me enough to unpack.

# [ 69 ]

# AN ODE TO ALL THE WAYS I'VE LEFT MY BODY

The next layer of gratitude I'm going to share is often elusive. It's the destination I've only found when I do the scary and often gut-wrenching work of inviting my protectors in for tea.

Now, my "managers" are often pretty comfortable being invited in, sharing some tea and over-eating biscuits with me. *They especially love the elephant shaped ones with white icing.* Many of the "managers" are familiar with logical conversations and using the spoken word for communication. They are pretty well-versed in making the rational case for how they're trying to protect me. It doesn't mean they're always eager to put down their armor, but the conversations are often pretty straightforward.

My "firefighters", on the other hand, are a lot harder to nail down. Because they don't use words or logic to protect me. They're sneaky at disguising their ~~destructive~~ protective behaviors. **Especially my *Fire Captain.***

My internal fire department's captain is *Miss Dissociation.* And she makes it nearly impossible to have a conversation with her.

> I'll often get a glimpse of her walking up to my house, so I'll head over to open the door - trying to be an attentive host. But in the 5 seconds it takes for me to walk there, she's gone and I'm left confused as to why I just opened the door to an empty space.
>
> I'll continue cleaning, listening to a podcast - then I'll hear the doorbell. I'll walk over to the door again. And again, I'm left standing on an empty threshold, wondering how I got there.
>
> By the time I can wrangle her into the sunroom, it takes me ten times as long as it should to make the tea because my mind loses track of what it was doing. I get distracted. I do a little more cleaning, I go read a few chapters in my book, I eat lunch, I go get the mail.
>
> It's not until I inadvertently walk into the sunroom again after running errands that I remember she's waiting for me. And when I go to fetch her tea, it's cold. And I start the process all over again...

You see, I didn't realize my standard operating procedure in life was dissociation until my late twenties.

The necessary perspective to see how far gone I was from my body - is the same perspective I was severed from.

It's hard for a floating head to know they're a floating head.

The part of me that used dissociation for protection seemed to have a never-ending supply of ways to actually accomplish this disconnection...

**Miss Dissociation's Toolbox Included:**

- Fantasy/Daydreaming
- Watching TV to zone out
- Playing through injury (*mind over matter, ya'll*)
- Staying busy all the time
- Alcohol
- Pain pills
- Leaving my body during sex
- Over-working
- "Vacation-scrolling"
- Travel*

**That last one was really hard to admit. Sometimes I used travel to connect to myself and enjoy time off from work. Other times, Miss Dissociation lured me in - with country counting and escapism.*

---

It took a great deal of patience and persistence to have meaningful conversations with *Miss Dissociation*. But gradually over time, she revealed more of herself to me. Microscopic bits at first.

The trust formed slowly over time. **As trust after rupture often does.**

I would sit for hours having "conversations" with my body. She didn't communicate with words. So I learned to speak *her* language. Making space for her to share through sensations, movement, tears, and primal sounds.

I'd listen, even when I didn't understand. *Especially when I didn't understand.*

Eventually... something started to shift...

The frustration, hopelessness, and sense of betrayal I used to feel towards *Miss Dissociation* began to morph into something else. She was no longer the enemy I had to *pretend* to like so I could trick her into going away.

I *actually* started to like her.

Genuine understanding for her emerged. Compassion began to burst through my eyes when I'd sit with her. I finally got it. I understood *who* she'd been protecting all these years. It finally made sense to me why she'd been working so hard my entire life.

And FUUUUUUUUCK, had she ever been working hard.

She'd been working tirelessly - at a thankless job - for well over two decades.

She. Was. Exhausted.

And I couldn't blame her. The genuine gratitude I had for her pouring out of my eyes allowed everything she'd ever done to make sense. I connected the dots. I apologized for all the terrible things I'd said about her over the years.

She wasn't broken. She wasn't a lost cause. **She was my biggest protector when I had none.**

I thanked her for protecting me. Over and over, I thanked her.

---

This relationship with *Miss Dissociation* transformed my life. Understanding, loving, and trusting each other fundamentally changed everything.

She began to see me as an adult. Not just in age - but as a wise, competent adult that she could trust.

She realized for the first time that it actually *wasn't* her job to keep me safe.

She didn't need to work so hard anymore.

She could finally rest.

And trust *me* to take care of things.

## [ 70 ]

# PASS THE BATON

I like to image the different parts of myself throughout my life are like a relay team. When I actually got to know *Miss Dissociation,* I learned how much she'd been trying to keep me safe me whole life.

It's not about getting rid of her now.

It's about letting her know she's already finished her leg of the race. And now, it's safe to pass the baton to me. I can take it from here.

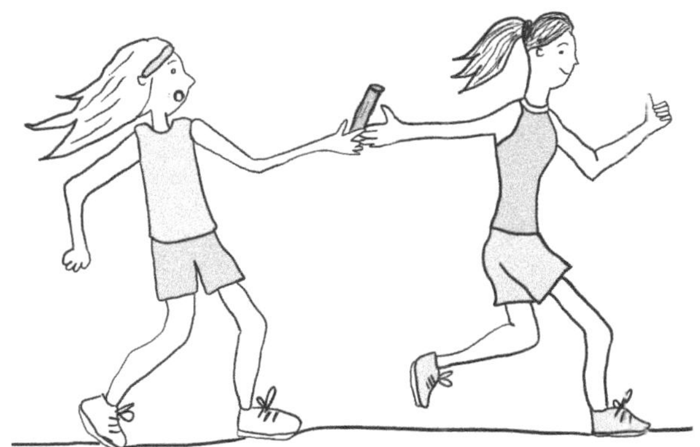

## [ 71 ]

## "BURN IT ALL DOWN"

Here's a little more context to the *"Burn it all down!"* message that Mama Shroom delivered shortly after closing down my therapy practice. This inner ~~whisper~~ yeller hinted that maybe it wasn't *just* my individual work with clients that needed to end.

Of course, I tried to talk myself out of this. I put blinders on and tried to use logic with the messenger. I rationalized that closing down all of my groups was a bit extreme.

*"How would I replace my income without the retreats?"* I bargained.

Then, the messenger tried to make a final point. One that was familiar from a mere few months prior. The same words that had convinced me to close my therapy practice.

> *"You can choose to work WITH the universe and end this on your terms. Or, it'll be done for you... but it won't be on your terms.*

But this time, I didn't listen. I pretended the 'check engine' light *didn't* just come on. *And we all know from the "Failure" chapter what happened next with Adventure Club.*

I wanted the *"Burn it all down!"* messages to be "too harsh" or "too extreme". I wanted it to be a metaphor gone wrong. *Oh hey there, wishful thinking.*

But I'm not so sure it was.

It's the difference between a prescribed burn and a wildfire.

And because of my unwillingness to burn the necessary acreage for protection, the flames ignited and I lost control over when and how it spread. I lost control over when and how these groups ended.

And then, I noticed there were even more aspects of my life affected by the fires. Areas of my life I'd tried to avoid in the Spring. Beyond just career, work, and business - it also started to impact some of my most sacred personal relationships.

This is where I *really* started resisting. Fighting against reality. Not wanting to acknowledge what was happening. Partially because, I naively thought I was done with that part of life. At least for a little while. The part of life I'd already navigated after my divorce, characterized by massive relationship evolution.

> Family becoming strangers.
>
> Strangers becoming family.

I *wanted* to be done - with all of it.

And, once again, I could see wishful thinking as the charismatic and persuasive protector of my psyche that she is. While also knowing - she is no match for reality.

**The hard truth about becoming the next version of who you're meant to be is that not everyone you love will come with you.**

People that were your entire world in one season of life will become unknown to you in the next. If evolution and reinvention is part of your path as an individual, it makes sense that your relationships will also change and adjust to the new reality of life.

A weekend trip to the city where my adult life and therapy career began proved to be the catalyst for even more shedding. More burning. More letting go and trusting that the void left behind - is necessary.

The inner message was clear:

*What you're meant to create from the void - isn't possible without it.*

## [ 72 ]

# "MARIE KONDO" YOUR LIFE

"A dramatic reorganization of the home causes correspondingly dramatic changes in lifestyle and perspective. It is life transforming."
-Marie Kondo, The Life-Changing Magic of Tidying Up

This is typically a practice I encourage people to do in the Spring. Clearing out and decluttering your life to create space for what's to come. But we're not always ready, in March, for the deep layers of *Radical Honesty* required for this kind of exercise.

I know I wasn't.

I held onto relationships, social media followers, past ideas about what my business should be, and an outdated wardrobe.

But returning home from my weekend trip, I knew what I needed to do.

I could no longer run from the fact that life was changing. And the life I wanted to create, both personally and professionally, was only possible by being in the void for a while.

The mud before the lotus.

The ashes before the rising.

And my path to create the life I desired, led me down the familiar hallway to an *Empty Room.*

Except the room wasn't empty yet. *That* was the part I still needed to do.

The practices to *Know Yourself* are never done. Every time you evolve into a new version of yourself, you have an opportunity to get to know the "new you".

And one way to do this is through creating an *Empty Room.*

**Literally and Metaphorically.**

By channeling the life-changing magic of taking your life apart, in order to put it back together in ways that make more sense.

Here's how it looked like for me in *this* chapter of my life...

**Literally:**

- End the one remaining group I was still holding onto.
- Stop planning for in-person retreats at the end of the year.
- Remove hundreds of social media followers.
- Delete email subscribers.
- Decluttering exercises in my home.
- Send the gut-wrenching email that confirms a hard ending.

**Metaphorically:**

- Reflect on every single relationship in my life.
- Imagine the *Empty Room* relationally - it's just me, alone in the room.

Once I created my *Empty Room*, I let the frosty air of discomfort seep through the cracks in the window as I sat in the potential of the dark and vast void.

With the cold, hard floor underneath me, I remained tethered to the possibility on the other side of this particular discomfort. Remembering the first time I "Marie Kondo'd" my life...

Almost a decade before this moment, I didn't have muscle memory built up yet. My discernment muscles were weak the first time I tried to "tidy up" my life.

The big, life-changing decisions hadn't happened overnight. But I guess you could still call it **"magic"** if you define magic as consistently listening to yourself and making aligned choices - *even* when they disappoint people. And working really hard to create the life you desire - *even* when it means ending relationships, jobs, and old patterns that aren't serving you anymore.

> **If "magic" = doing the things that scare you most because you know they're right. Then yes, Marie Kondo's book was magic. And life-changing.**

I hold on to that memory now. A beacon of hope as once again the world swirls around me. Part of me: scared and uncertain. Another part: confident from years of *Radical Honesty* and *Know Yourself* practices.

And then...

I slowly and deliberately begin to fill the *Empty Room*.

One relationship and one throw pillow at a time.

With only what makes sense in my life, *now*.

## [ 73 ]

## "I CAN'T WAIT TO SEE WHAT HAPPENS IN OCTOBER INSTEAD."

When I decided to close my therapy practice, I needed *something* to grasp on to. Anything really. Anything I could use to justify to myself why I was essentially taking a torch to the financial security I'd only recently become accustomed to.

I definitely entertained the part of me who suggested that closing my practice was an act of self-sabotage because I wasn't used to abundance. This part told me I'd reached my upper limit financially and was trying to regulate back to the place of having "just enough" that I was so familiar with.

This *was* a good point and something to consider. It might've even been true for someone else. But it wasn't the full picture for me.

That's the thing about the internal family. The different parts often wear blinders. They have limited perspective and can only see the thing they've been trained to be hyper-focused on. They are limited to the mindset they had at the age they became "stuck".

Self is the one who's able to zoom out and have perspective. To listen to *all* the voices. And it was Self's voice (*my voice*) I heard whispering to me back in early July...

> *"I can't wait to see what happens in October instead..."*

This steady and wise inner voice knew that the "failure" I was in the middle of wasn't the full picture. Self knew there was something different meant for me in the fall. And it wasn't possible to have both. This "failure" was necessary in order to make space for something even bigger.

**Trusting yourself doesn't mean you have all the answers, all the time.**

While I was in a state of shock and fear, realizing that the rest of the year wouldn't look the way I'd predicted, Self didn't jump in and tell me exactly *how* it would change for the better. Instead, Self just planted the seed that settled my entire body by hinting there might be something unexpected coming in October.

There's often more at play than we can see close up. But when you have a strong sense of trust in yourself, you're able to see the magic in the blindside. Maybe even see it as divine redirection from Self.

---

It's October now. And as I sit here and write the words in the book you're reading, I'm also in the middle of launch week for my first book - "The 13 Lessons" book.

I'm not doing any of what *"June Emily"* dreamed of and predicted. I'm not in Southern California running a beautiful

Alumni Retreat for all three seasons of *Adventure Club*. Season 3 didn't even happen. None of what I held onto as a life raft in order to have the courage to close my practice happened. None of what I *thought* I wanted - happened.

Instead, I'm Self-publishing a book. With all the capital-S, "Self energy" I can access. I'm surrendering to the magic of this blindside.

And I'm writing words I never thought I'd say back in July...

**"I'm really grateful no one signed up."**

[ 74 ]

# BIRTH RITUALS

In the psychedelic chapter at the beginning of the book, I encouraged you to think about ways to have a mystical or psychedelic experience *without* ingesting anything.

Because remember: this approach does *not* require you to take any substances to benefit from the medicine that is: *intentional ritual.*

I'm frequently reminded of what my psychedelic therapy mentor, *Lauren Taus*, says:

> *"Life is psychedelic. Integration is a lifestyle."*

I put this concept into practice in the days leading up to the birth of my first book. I wanted to bring ceremony to this moment in time. To ritualize the threshold from writer to author.

Advanced planning can be helpful for rituals like this. I was able to set myself up to have no commitments for almost two days. An entire weekend for the birth portal. And when the morning arrived, I was grateful to my *Past Self* for arranging everything.

The portal opened by having an energy and body work session. I'd been working with my practitioner for many years by this point. The trust had been long established and I'd had many experiences to know that she was capable of holding space for anything that arose in session - physically, emotionally, logistically, or spiritually - in any realm. She incorporates many modalities into her work but has a special emphasis on the womb - the space for creation. The metaphor for birth blended beautifully with the work she does every day in the literal birth space.

As with actual psychedelic experiences, it's often difficult to put words to the experience. Synesthiesia is also common. This is a phenomenon that can feel like the wires to your senses get crossed. You can taste colors and feel sounds. You can have an experience of everything making sense while simultaneously nothing makes any sense all. Paradox prevails. You can feel intense and profound emotions that are impossible to explain logically.

Fueled by intention, silence, breathwork, music, and the physical touch from Sydney - this session became the birthing space. Three hours later, I left the session with a sense of clarity, calm, and confidence about the next chapter I was walking into.

> Preparation - *check*
>
> Mystical experience - *check*
>
> Then, it was time for integration...

Integration looks a lot like self care. And just like caring for yourself on a consistent basis, integration of healing experiences often requires being very deliberate. You have to find a way to keep it at the forefront of your mind or it can be tempting to fall back into routines of disconnection and auto-pilot living.

The first 48-72 hours following a psychedelic journey is a particularly important window for integration practices as the brain is in a highly malleable state. This allows the brain to be more receptive to change and forming new neural pathways.

This is a visual representation of how many more parts of your brain are able to communicate during and after a psilocybin (magic mushroom) experience, but results are similar with other non-ordinary states of consciousness. Many new pathways are created.

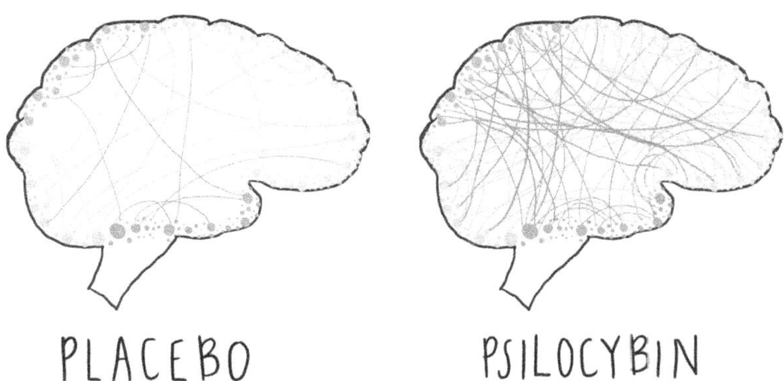


**Here are some practical ways to help integrate any type of transformative experience:**

- Reduce media input.
- Nature: reconnect with nature and allow yourself to experience 'awe'.

- Movement: connect to your body through yoga, hiking, Tai Chi, dance, drumming, etc.
- Music: listen to the music from your journey or other nature sounds.
- Journal: reflect and write about your experience.
    - What do you remember?
    - What clarity did you find?
    - A personal favorite integration prompt of mine: *How can I keep the gifts I received in my journey alive in my daily life?*
- Art: create art inspired by your journey.
- Connect: share your experience with your support system and other people who "get it".
- Pay attention to your dreams afterwards.
- Care for your body: eat nourishing foods, rest, take a relaxing bath.

It's this final bullet point that became my to-do list for the rest of the day. And with my proclivity for the hard work part of this process, I knew it would be a challenge.

But a challenge worth exploring.

---

The next morning I filled my hiking daypack with one extra item. *My debut book.*

"The 13 Lessons" was coming with me on the aspen lined trails.

The tiny yellow leaves I was surrounded by reminded me what I was ready to let go of, while also connecting me to a sense of awe, wonder, and appreciation.

There was an abundance of gratitude. With each step, reflecting on everything that had gotten me to that point. And readying myself for harvest.

The visuals from the previous day's bodywork session filled my mind.

I eventually found a large rock to rest on - half in the sun, half in the shade. I sat down to try and put words to the ineffable experience I'd had the day before. Attempting to capture the essence so I could return to it - when *Future Me* might need the medicine most.

> **I wrote about who I hoped my book would reach.**
>
> **I wrote about the impact I hoped it would have.**
>
> **I wrote about what I hoped I could open myself up to by publishing it.**

And then I wrote a letter.

Apparently *Future Me* already has the wisdom from the medicine.

> Dear Em,
>
> You're on the cusp of something really fucking cool.
>
> Tomorrow - is simultaneously just another Sunday and also... a pivotal threshold for you.
>
> You will be a published author. Seriously. An *actual* author. It's kind of a big deal. And

also, not far from now, this new aspect of your identity will start to feel normal.

You'll soon be able to introduce yourself as an author with as much confidence as you've responded, "I'm a therapist", for over a decade.

I know this next part is going to be hard for you - but I really want you to try and ENJOY the moment. Stretch your capacity to receive the excitement, joy, and people feeling inspired.

Don't rush past this part just because you're uncomfortable. Soak it in.

And trust.

Trust that the right people will be magnetized to it. This book *will* find its way to the people it's meant for.

Sometimes this will happen by you getting uncomfortable and talking about it.

Sometimes the universe will do the work for you - and you'll have no idea how someone found it.

Both paths are important. Trust in both.

There are things you can (and will have to) do to help this book find its people.

AND.

There's some magic to all of this.

I'm not sure if I should tell you this or not, but I'm going to. This won't be your only book. You have many more books in you. I know that feels unimaginable right now. But I promise you - it happens. It really does.

And you'll feel different with each new book release. They will all be special in their own way.

But you will never publish your *first* book again.

This moment - is it.

I know you're more comfortable rushing ahead to the next thing (I get it, so am I).

But please, I beg of you. Be present with your first.

This is the book that makes you an author.

Cherish her. Cherish it. Give the reverence you preach.

Tomorrow - you'll be an author. I'll see you on the other side...

with love and clarity,
5x bestselling author - Emily Romero

I don't know when the future version of myself will be a 5x bestselling author or if she's a-lot-a-bit delusional. Is this letter from a version of me 10 years in the future, or 50?

After re-reading the letter in my journal now, I have serious doubts if it will ever happen. But that's the wondrous thing about letters from your *Future Self*.

**It's not logic who writes them**.

When I do this practice I try to reach that liminal headspace that isn't filled with rational static. I sit down and let the words flow onto the page from something beyond me in that present moment.

Whatever happens now, happens.

The book is birthed... And now, I try to let go of any attachment to a specific outcome.

## [ 75 ]

# INNER CHILD WORK

Speaking of different versions of yourself, we've talked about your *Future Self* quite a bit in this book already, but what about your *Past Self*? There are many powerful practices that strengthen the relationship with the younger versions of you.

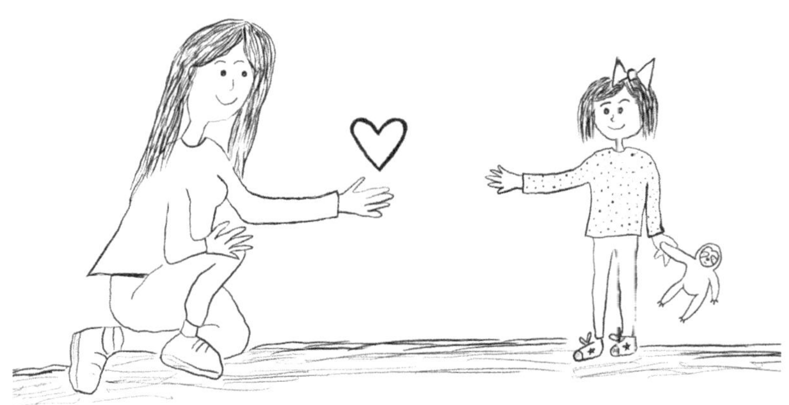

**Here are a few ideas to get you started thinking about how to nurture these relationships inside:**

- Look through photos of you from the past.
    - Connect to her, talk to her, appreciate her.
- Frame a photo of younger you.
    - Find a photo of yourself that feels resonate when you look at it.
    - Display it in a place where you can see it daily.
    - Commit to connecting to her daily for six months, even if it's just a quick "hello".
- Do things your younger parts loved to do.
    - Take her on a play date to do all her favorite things... get ice cream, go roller skating, watch her favorite movie, etc.
    - Let her choose.
- Write letters to/from all the different versions of yourself.
    - Gratitude from *Current You* to a past version that made a really difficult decision.
    - Letter from *Future You* with words of wisdom and advice as you navigate through a challenging time - *like my book birthing letter*.
- Dominant/Non-Dominant Hand Writing
    - Open you notebook so you have two blank pages side by side.
    - Using your dominant hand, write as *Current You.* Asking for guidance from *Future You.*
    - Using your non-dominant hand, answer the questions as *Future You.*
    - Continue the conversation back and forth between *Current You* and *Future You.*

## [ 76 ]
## AUTHOR-IN-TRAINING

My first published book is short.

A couple months before publication, my husband and I were at a local bookstore conducting a little research. Looking at book covers to see which ones caught our eye.

I picked up a small blue cover and flipped through the pages, quickly landing at the back.

**124 pages.**

I scoff and ask him, *"Do you think this guy calls himself an author?"*

With a slightly confused look, he responds definitively, *"Yes, I do."*

My insecurity-based projection onto a successful author I don't even know mirrors the relentless questioning in my mind recently.

- *Can I even call it a book if it's less than 150 pages?*

- *Can I call myself an author?*

Frequently, my answer to both questions is "*No.*"

But luckily, I don't let that be the final answer. Thankfully, I've gained another perspective I can counter with, that also happens to feel true most days.

This first part of this perspective shift is realized when I remember that my book used to be nearly twice as long. And just because the first draft was much longer, did not make it better. In fact, it was messy, confusing, and disorganized. *That's what I get for trying to cram 35 lessons into 13.*

Simply stated, by cutting out what was unnecessary, the book got better.

**The length of the book does not necessarily correlate to the impact of the book.**

I also remember how that first book is serving the bigger picture in many indirect ways. I'm getting on the job training - with 114 pages instead of 468. I get to tighten the loop on every stage of the process and learn more quickly through trial and error.

> *Less money spent on editing.*
>
> *Lower printing costs.*
>
> *Less time recording the audio version.*

I'm learning how to Self-publish a book by *doing* it.

Also, I get to close the therapist chapter of my life, officially. And I get to stretch myself in the most uncomfortable ways and begin being more visible. I get to begin sharing my writing and taking up space - with a book that is markedly less vulnerable than what I eventually want to share.

It's about titration. Remembering how important *Regulation* is.

I'm transitioning from sporadic journaler → writer → author in a way that won't overwhelm my nervous system and send me running back to the safe anonymity of the therapist chair.

# [ 77 ]
# HEROIC DOSE OF MY OWN MEDICINE

In the early chapter on "Dosing", I introduced you to the term "heroic dose". This is a term coined by *Terence McKenna* to capture a particularly high dose of dried psilocybin mushrooms that leads to the ***ego death/"I'm a changed person"/life-altering kind of journey*** described by plant medicine evangelists.

> *PS. This approach isn't for most people. But now you have context.*

Recently, I was asked about the biggest lessons I've learned since beginning this Self-publishing journey. And even though I've been applying *The Self-Trust Model* to my life for many years and directly to my business during the writing of this book, deciding to publish a book ramped *everything* up.

You've had a chance, by now, to hear how *Doubt* has shown up in my life. While she's much less influential in my decision making process than she once was, she still, very much, wants to be heard.

Here's a truth that might be confronting to hear:

**Building Self-Trust does not mean *Doubt* gets kicked out of your internal family.**

Quite the opposite. Remember, the IFS approach is not about eliminating protective parts. Instead, cultivating more trust in myself has pushed me into arenas I never would've been in before. Even just a few years ago, I never would've allowed myself to publish a book or tell people I wrote a book or pause everything else in my business to market a book.

It would've been too vulnerable. Too risky. Too scary. Too uncertain. Too much possibility that I'd fail. Or worse yet, I might be misunderstood.

So my answer to what is my biggest lesson so far in publishing a book?

**Sharing it with the world often requires taking a heroic dose of your own medicine.**

So of course, since my work is all about Self-Trust and trusting your intuition, *this* is what's being tested in me.

*Doubt* has gotten very loud over the past couple of months. Not because this whole Self-Trust thing doesn't work, but because it does. The work I've done for a decade to build trust in myself is now putting me in situations that have blasted me out of my comfort zone. Blasted me into the ***ego death/"I'm a changed person"/life-altering kind of journey.***

Over and over again, I have to return to the Self-Trust practices I teach:

- I have to get **Radically Honest** with myself about if this path is still what I want and WHY it's worth it.
- I have to set commitments from Self energy - and then, **Keep** my **Promises**.
- I have to check in with my body, nurture her, and prioritize practices that encourage **Regulation** in my nervous system.
- I have to remember who the fuck I am. I have to get to **Know Myself**, over and over again, through each evolution.

## [ 78 ]

## PENELOPE ROSE & CHERYL

Now that my first book is published and available for people to find, buy, read, misunderstand, rip to shreds, project their stuff onto, or maybe even, enjoy, I'm discovering I now have two distinct jobs. Jobs that are so divergent in their roles, they need different names.

First up, is **Penelope Rose**. That's a mouthful so she goes by "PR" for short.

PR does what you might expect from her "Public Relations" initials. She is in charge of waking up first thing in the morning, and before she's even out of bed - checking the dashboard to see how many books were purchased while we were sleeping. Then she checks the email provider website to see if there were any new subscribers. She does the same for social media. Then, it's time to check the book listing page to see if any new reviews came through. She screenshots any good ones and logs them into the spreadsheet.

*Yes, PR has even forced me to overcome my aversion to spreadsheets. Maybe people can change...*

Then, she looks in the folder labeled: *Viral Marketing Ideas,* to see if in a prior moment of inspiration, she'd created any fantastic viral content about the book. If not (*it's always, not*) she looks at a blank page and tries to come up with some clever marketing strategy on the fly that will sell hundreds of copies. Then she curses, *"Stupid fucking videos on the internet."* All of this, before getting camera ready for a podcast interview because everyone now insists on video for the formerly audio-only media.

PR doesn't feel particularly good at her job. But she's trying. And every time she gets a hit of dopamine seeing another book sale, she decides she can wait another day before putting in her two-week notice.

PR's favorite time of the day, though, is when she gets to clock out. Of course, in typical PR fashion, she has a hard time *actually* clocking out. Clicking "refresh" a couple more times on the book sales dashboard before she *finally* logs out. She doesn't have great work/life boundaries. But I need her to. So Cheryl can get to work.

You see, **Cheryl** is the writer. And yes, Cheryl was named after a grief-stricken through-hiker who captured her pain in her memoir, *Wild,* a couple of decades ago. Cheryl doesn't have to worry about what people think of her writing. Cheryl doesn't waste time ruminating on what *User45924* said about her first book. She's mastered the art of not giving a fuck. Cheryl expects to be misunderstood and thinks she's probably not doing her job very well if everyone likes her. Plus, she cracks herself up with jokes she knows will be removed in the editing process, but writes them anyway.

Cheryl tries not to think about PR too much. She knows they're colleagues and they should try to get along. But she doesn't want PR's political correctness to wear off on her, so she keeps her distance. Sometimes she even tries to sneak a little "trojan horse" into the writing that PR will have to try to explain later.

As their manager, one thing I've learned is PR and Cheryl can't work together. I have to put them on different shifts. Even though they each understand why I keep the other one around, I got tired of breaking up fights between them.

This is an example of internal family members who are better able to love each other - *from afar*.

[ 79 ]

# AN EARLY FREEZE

October 25th

Post-launch depression is real.

Even though we're just beginning to reach idealistic fall temperatures here in Denver, my "personal season" has already rushed ahead to the cold and frigid days of winter.

I poured everything I had into making my book a reality. I put everything else aside (even the things that actually make my business money) to focus on this one project. For months, I was fueled by adrenaline and anticipation. And the fear that my savings wouldn't last as long as I budgeted for.

All leading me to "launch day"... which turned

into "launch week"... which is now turning into "launch month".

And now, I'm fucking exhausted.

All I want to do is channel my inner hyber-nating grizzly and never talk to another podcast host. I never want to make another social media post enticing people to immediately go "buy my book!"

And I definitely don't want to stand in front of a group of strangers reading words in public... that I wrote in private.

Just like certain snowy winter days, right now it feels like this freeze will never pass. It feels like it will be this way forever.

Cold and lonely. Tired and dark. A part of me wants to hibernate forever. She is very convincing with her hot mug of tea, oversized blankets, and Hallmark movies.

Her presence, though, doesn't keep me from also remembering that every single winter I've ever experienced has eventually thawed.

I just don't know when...

[ 80 ]

# PERSPECTIVE IN THE MOMENT

I've never been in the throes of hardship or navigating acute pain and thought to myself, *"I'm so grateful I'm going through this! Yay, now I'll be able to normalize this for someone else later!"*

In fact, I've often found grief and depression to be a very self-centered experienced. I don't really have capacity to think about how my current reality might be able to help others in the future. It feels irrelevant when I'm not sure if I'll even make it through the storm.

Now, my experience of post-launch depression is not completely debilitating. I'm not going to sit here and pretend that the kind of perspective I'm about to talk about is possible during everyone's darkest nights of the soul. In fact, I think it's a requirement to actively question if you'll even survive most dark nights.

**And survival mode... is not conducive to meaning making.**

But my post launch experience is somewhere in-between. There are definitely moments of:

- *"What the fuck did I just do?"*
- *"Now what?"*
- *"Did I just waste a bunch of time and money… for nothing?"*

There are days when I sit and stare at my computer screen, willing *Penelope Rose* to come up with something clever to post. But she just stares back at me - doe eyed and confused. There are moments when my arms feel like sandbags, so I decide it's a better option to just stay in bed, look at the back of my eyelids, and remember how great it used to feel when I was financially secure. I even let myself fantasize briefly about having a stable 9-5 job. *Ooo La La.*

I allow fear to drag me down some catastrophizing rabbit holes. And even though I stopped drinking years ago, my hangovers are back with a vengeance. Who knew being visible online was way worse than ten Captain & Ginger Ales? I develop a new respect for social media influencers while secretly wondering, *"Are they really okay?"*

What I'm experiencing does NOT feel sustainable. It's not fun, I don't *enjoy* it.

But I've also experienced enough life to have some perspective. No one is dead or dying. My savings will last until I figure out my next move.

The aftermath of launching *is* hard. Just as the hard of doing anything new is hard. But it's a doable hard. It's a "hard" I would choose again. And it's a "hard" that I can now provide perspective on, for someone else.

Since I began sharing with others that I wrote a book, I've lost count of the number of people who've told me it's also a dream of theirs - a dream they've "never told anyone else."

*Uh oh, am I slipping back into familiar therapy territory?*

They tell me about the story (or stories) that are living in them that they want to share with the world. I hear how liberating they imagine the book writing process to be - immediately followed by all the reasons they haven't done it yet. I'm invited to their "parts party" for a little bit.

So, even in the midst of my hangovers and emotional spirals, I'm still tethered to the perspective that my current reality will be helpful for others. I understand that I'm actively experiencing things that I can share with other writers who claim themselves as "not a writer". And when they cross the threshold to becoming an author, I can normalize the "parts party" that ensues and the incessant and addicting pattern of clicking "refresh" on the book sales dashboard.

For the first time, I can understand in the moment, how my current challenges are going to be a beacon of hope for someone else. And in some ways, that makes it worth it.

[ 81 ]

# "OPPOSITE OF A SELF-HELP BOOK!"

I eventually accepted that the trail I was on - happened to be the author path. And once I did this, I couldn't help but think about the books that had changed my life. And how many times I've felt surges of gratitude for the women brave enough to put their stories on paper.

The vulnerable and gritty memoir authors. I dreamed that one day I could be as courageous as they are.

But somehow, the first two books I wanted to write seemed to be in the genre of self-help, instead of the dark and twisty memoir. So, I questioned myself:

> *Did I really want to be a part of the multi-billion dollar self-help world that sometimes causes more harm than good?*

No, not really... but also... *these* were the books I wanted to write first.

Thankfully, one of the first pieces of feedback I received about my first book emboldened me to continue. Because even though

I clearly lay out "The 13 Lessons" from my time as a therapist in that book - her feedback spoke to the tone and message underneath.

**"It's like the opposite of a self-help book!"**

She went on to tell me how she was left with a sense of being more connected to *herself* after reading. She didn't feel like she was being prescribed... *anything*. Other than to listen to her own wisdom. And now she had a lot of jumping off points to do that.

My intention for the book was coming through... at least to one person. And it inspired me to keep going. All the way to this book. The one you're holding in your hands now. Which you very well could've found in the self-help section of your library. But, if it is in fact a self-help book...

**It's a self-help book for people who don't like being told what to do.**

# [ PART 4 ]
# WINTER

We restore... with the essence of the **Winter Solstice.**

A retreat inward.

A time to rest after Fall's harvest.

A symbolic death of ego and identity.

A cozy day snuggled up with a warm cup of tea, a good book, and the softest blanket.

An introspective reflection on life lived.

A liminal space and slower pace.

A loving embrace with the medicine of darkness.

Bringing completion to this cycle of your life...

Honoring goodbyes with reverence...

The period on the final page...

. . .

And eventually, we prepare for the next Spring.

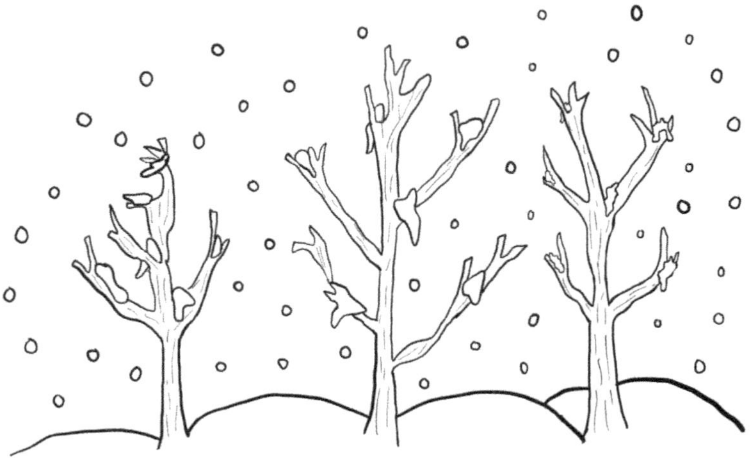

## [ 82 ]

# WINTERING

December 21st

I've had this undeniable urge to "nest" for a while. I don't even fully know what I mean when I say that, but it's just the word that won't leave me alone.

I just want to NEST. (And no, I'm not pregnant.)

I also decided to get off social media. To actually delete it from my phone. This is counter to every "business coach" I've ever listened to. But in all honesty, I'm feeling pretty skeptical of all business coaches right now. Especially if they built their business solely by helping others grow a business.

I know I've been saying all year that I want to "slow down" and "pause" and "rest". And I havent always done a very good job at it. Okay, MOST of the time, I havent done a good job at it.

But this time feels... different.

I'm at some sort of threshold. Some kind of tipping point.

But today has given me a lot of compassion for my "Hardworking Part". I get it, a little bit more, why she's had such a death grip on my life.

All day - I've had this existential, deep feeling of "what's the point of any of this?"

It went dark - fast.

And then I felt these two conflicting messages arise. One on each shoulder - but I dont think either one is the angel.

Message 1: You're just a victim of capitalism. We all are! You've been conditioned your entire life to value productivity, money, and achievement above all else. Rest is how you liberate yourself! The only way to fix yourself is to become one with your couch!

Message 2: Resting is uncomfortable AF. You know how to make the discomfort go away... just produce an offering to sell. Or start taking 1-1 clients again. Or honestly, just create a completely unnecessary to-do list so you can stay busy all day. The only way to fix yourself is to do more.

Yep, I think I've got devils on both shoulders.

Here's all I know right now:

- I know the pull in me to "nest" and to "winter" is real.
- I know becoming one with my couch isn't the answer.
- I know creating an unnecessary to-do list, also, isn't the answer.
- I know there are parts of me craving to be seen and known in this process of nesting.
- I know there is something big waiting for me inside the discomfort.
- I know this isn't a "quick win" situation.
- I know I want to create - more than I produce.
- I know my impact matters.
- And, I know I'll know more... eventually.

## [ 83 ]
## THE WORLD CONSPIRES

Sometimes the metaphorical seasons of our life align with the actual season happening in nature all around us.

And sometimes - they don't.

Sometimes, you'll go through a painful summer breakup. Or you'll get laid off right as the cherry blossoms offer a promise of new life. Or your dog (*who's so much more than just a dog*) will die just as everyone else is celebrating a season of gratitude.

Sometimes the misalignment can feel cruel.

The incongruence from what we're experiencing in life compared to the expectations of the season can feel unbearable.

I've found it's most helpful to honor the *internal* season. To be honest with myself about the season I'm *actually* in - regardless of what the leaves may or may not be doing outside.

While I felt the "early freeze" after my book launch, I didn't honor it for long. I allowed a day of "recovery" and then set my sights on the next goal. I moved the finish line... again.

I told myself - after my book signing event - *then*, I'll rest.

No part of me was surprised by how drained I was at the end of the night of this event. The never-ending flow from one conversation to another. Catching up with people I hadn't seen in years. Trying hard not to deflect words of praise and congratulations. I collapsed into my bed that night with achy feet, a full heart, and a desire to not speak to anyone for a month.

The universe tried to help me with my seasonal confusion. I returned home and the temperatures dropped from sunny and 80 degrees to a dreary 40. It felt like the liminal week between Christmas and New Year's - even though it wasn't quite Halloween. My period even started early - the winter of the menstrual cycle. Everything was conspiring to push me into rest. The outside trying to match my inside.

I didn't have any good excuses to keep working.

**So why is this still so hard?**

[ 84 ]

# FAKING IT

If you would've asked me while I was working as a therapist how much of my identity, worth, or value was related to that job title, I would've shrugged and responded, "*Not much*".

And I wouldn't have been trying to lie to you. But the lie to myself - apparently ran deep.

---

"*So, what do you do?*"

It wasn't until I awkwardly stumbled over my words trying to answer this question from a stranger that I realized how much I still had to learn about these parts inside me.

The part that tightly coupled my identity with my work.

And the best way that she knew to eliminate any discomfort – was to work harder. "Rest" was a plague to avoid.

---

But this was a lesson I thought I'd already learned. I'd sat with *Miss Dissociation* for plenty of tea times by this point in life. *Hundreds* of tea times. This is partially what led to closing down my therapy practice in the first place.

I knew it wasn't just one of those *"hustle and grind"* seasons of business. Deep down, I knew I needed to actively choose to do less. I knew I could partner *with* the universe in a shared endeavor of rest - or I could wait and see how the lesson would be thrust upon me.

I needed to slow down, get curious, and be deliberate in my next steps. I knew that as familiar as over-working and staying busy all the time were to me, they weren't the answer now.

I saw through *Miss Dissociation*'s fear when she tried to convince me:

> *"Just keep doing it all a bit longer... you'll be fine!"*
>
> *"Once you make X amount of money or hit some other ambiguous milestone - then you can close your practice."*

I'd recognized her tactics right away. They were all too familiar by this point. I knew if I didn't take the leap to close my practice, there'd be a price to pay.

So... I listened.

I listened when my intuition told me to slow down.

I took action on the inconvenient truth.

I closed the part of my business that was my individual therapy practice. I quit working under my license. I did the hard thing! And damnit, I wanted a cookie for it! After all those years...

*I finally... learned how to rest.*

*I learned how to surrender.*

Except... and this probably comes as no surprise, I didn't. *It was all lies.*

*Miss Dissociation* had apparently upped her game. She'd learned to disguise herself even more. She'd gotten really good at convincing me I was taking a break.

*She convinced me I was taking a break by closing down my therapy practice...*

*She convinced me I was taking a break by pausing group events...*

But denial... is powerful.

And I wanted to believe her. I *wanted* to believe I'd finally learned to rest. If only so I could move on from that lesson and keep working.

But the only thing I'd learned to do was "fake surrender".

Unfortunately (or maybe fortunately) my body no longer lets me get away with telling lies to myself. The incongruence will always show up in my body.

And that's exactly what happened.

It was clearly time to head North again. Part of me was finally ready for the deeper layers of *Radical Honesty*.

Once again, radically honest reflection led to some very inconvenient truths about my life and business:

- The in-person event (*read: REALLY FUCKING GOOD IDEA!*) I started planning immediately after crossing the most recent "finish line" with my book, needed to be put on hold.
- The virtual end-of-year events I'd already planned also needed to wait.
- The 1-1 offer I *almost* started telling people about... you guessed it. Not the right time.
- The lesson for me was to learn what *true surrender* feels like. I couldn't keep pushing the finish line out if I wanted the life I claimed to.
- It was time to quiet the external noise.
- It was time to lean into winter. To follow my cravings for cozy, introspective, and spiritual practices.
- It was time for me to nest.

That's the word that kept coming in - nest. It wasn't "slow down", "do less", or even "take some time to rest".

The message was clear: *"It's time to nest."*

I didn't even really know what I meant when I said it. But I went ahead and shared the inner whisper with my husband. Saying it out loud allowed the truth of it to sink in.

Which activated my fear response.

It's like the moment in a mushroom journey when you realize where it might go - so you try to grasp on even tighter to avoid it. You try to clench control. You fight it. Screaming, *"I can't do this!!"* , becomes your mantra. Suffering prevails.

And then... finally... the "transition"... and you tip over... into ***true surrender***.

That's what it felt like... the grasping... the clenching... fighting my intuition... denying the inconvenient truth... bargaining with reality...

*Miss Dissociation* didn't want to nest. She was terrified of nesting. She wanted to go back to her old toolkit of staying busy. She was afraid of what would be required to truly surrender.

But she also knew - it was the only path forward.

## [ 85 ]

# DO THE OPPOSITE

I think this is as good of a time as any to enccurage you to NOT listen to anything I say. *Better than at the beginning of the book, eh?*

**I'm not an expert on your life.**

I have no idea what season of life you're in as you read this book. I have no idea what you've been through and what protective parts have formed because of it. I have no idea if you should quit your job or if you should become a mom or if you should move in with your girlfriend.

Those answers aren't in me.

But if you've been itching for some direct advice this whole book, I'm going to finally give it to you.

**Do the opposite of everything I've said so far.**

Pause. Bookmark this page. Do a little happy dance that you're off the hook.

Then, go back through the entire book and do the inverse of what I've shared.

- Lie to yourself.
- Flake on your commitments.
- Stay inside for weeks at a time.

Okay, okay... those ones I'm going to stand behind pretty firmly. I don't know a path to trusting yourself that is paved by lies and artificial light. But sometimes you have to learn that lesson for yourself - out of principle.

But I really do want you to think critically about some of the other exercises in this book. If there is an "opposite" path to explore - try it out. Allow yourself to get messy. Make "mistakes". Follow the pull inside - even if you can't discern yet if it's wishful thinking or your intuition.

Notice what *actually* resonates for you.

---

After a traumatic loss in my own life - I gave myself permission for one year to believe in all the signs and synchronicities I was experiencing. I gave myself permission to not doubt or diminish what I felt. I figured that at the end of the year, I'd either be grateful for the magical thinking that helped me survive the hardest thing I'd been through or I'd fundamentally have new beliefs about the human experience.

The following year, I gave myself permission to believe the exact opposite. To believe that nothing I'd felt or experienced over the past year was actually "true". That it was all just my mind trying to create connections to make death less painful.

I leaned in fully - both years. And where I landed on those beliefs about the human experience isn't really relevant. But the journey I took to get there is. And it's a path I encourage you to explore for yourself.

## [ 86 ]

# MANY PATHS; SAME DESTINATION

The first season of *Adventure Club* was spread out over six months. In addition to learning about the therapeutic frameworks that informed the model and navigating our way around the Self-Trust compass, each month, we also explored a different *Pathway to Self-Trust.*

A *Pathway to Self-Trust* is simple. It's anything you've already explored (or want to) that can support your goal of trusting yourself more. It's a way to take the intention for more Self-Trust and direct it into a single domain. While applying all four directions of the compass to it.

In that first season, we explored six of the pathways that had most supported my journey in Self-Trust. They included: solo travel, embodiment practices, exploring sexuality, use of psychedelics, hiking, and exploring spirituality.

As more and more women have applied this model to their own life, many other *Pathways to Self-Trust* have revealed themselves.

- Female friendships
- Waiting tables
- Becoming a step-parent
- Gardening
- Exploring *Human Design*
- Beekeeping
- Starting a business
- Learning *Feng Shui*
- Going to graduate school
- Conscious parenting
- Cooking
- Reiki training
- Weightlifting
- Trying a new sport as an adult
- Learning tarot
- Roller derby

This list is endless.

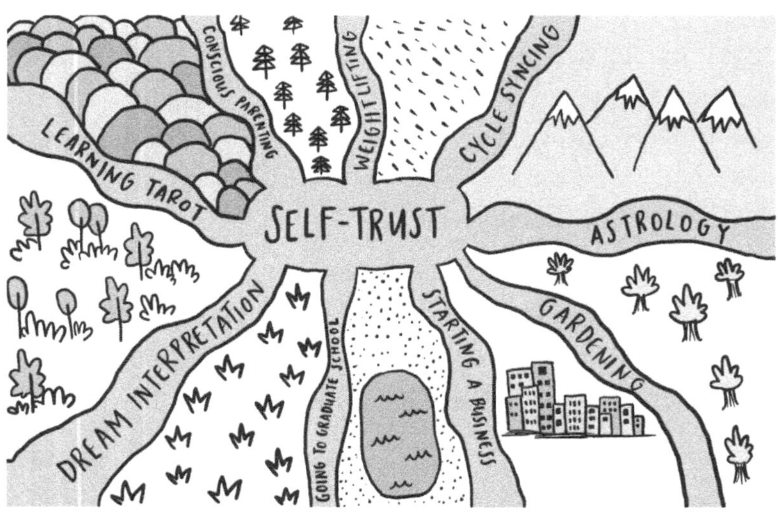

Notice if any of these pathways resonate with you. And then connect to your heart space and ask yourself:

- What pathways have I already explored?
- What have these pathways already taught me?
- What pathways am I curious to embark on?
- What pathways am I eager to travel down further?

## [ 87 ]

# SPIRITUAL AF

There's a good chance we'll all use different words to define "spiritual". It means different things to different people - depending on your *Life-Scripts* and the experiences you've had.

Some words that come to mind when I'm trying to explain my experience of the "woo-woo" are:

- The Mystery
- The Unknown
- The Sacred
- The Mystical
- The Unseen

**My definition of spirituality**: the practices that allow me to return home to myself, my body, my soul, my heart, and my connection with something beyond me.

This is why hiking in nature, eating mushrooms, moving my body, drinking tea, reading a book, journaling, listening to music, watching a sunrise or even having sex - *can be* spiritual practices for me. It comes back to the intention.

---

One of my favorite aspects of connecting one-on-one or working in small groups with people is the depth and nuance of conversations we get to explore.

And in my experience, spirituality is a realm that is best enjoyed together - with an open heart and an open mind.

I'm especially interested in how spiritual experiences and corresponding beliefs connect with Self-Trust.

- Are they related?
- Do they impact each other?

I once heard someone share her ideas around "something beyond" that really stuck with me.

And the beliefs she explained were simple - *we are all one.*

"Out there" we all began connected as one. The separation happened as we came into the human experience. But even as a human, we are all still part of that "oneness" of the beyond.

She went on to pose the idea that maybe "trusting the universe" - that oneness out there - is *actually* trusting yourself. Because you are a part of that whole.

And vice versa, when you build Self-Trust, it also deepens the trust you have in something beyond you. Whether you call that "something" - *The Divine, The Universe,* a higher power, God, Spirit, Allah, or just "something bigger than me".

This perspective challenged a view I'd had.

I'd often seen looking to a higher power for all the answers as a sign of lacking Self-Trust. It's often when we doubt ourselves the most, that we exasperatedly throw up our hands and say *"Universe, you decide for me!"*

But maybe it wasn't that simple...

---

I'm not ending this chapter with a conclusion about the "right" perspective. But, what I do hope you got from this chapter was an opportunity to react to external stimuli. To notice how *your* body responds to someone else's perspective. To illuminate *Life-Scripts* that may have impacted your beliefs. And I hope your response gave you more clarity about what *you* believe. And what you might be curious to explore more of.

## [ 88 ]

# A NOTE ON PERSONAL RESPONSIBILITY

At its most basic meaning, taking "personal responsibility" is *not* the idea that the things that have happened to you are your fault. But it *is* your responsibility in how you choose to move forward. It's also the idea that you get out what you put in. Instead of defaulting to blaming others and external circumstances.

And when you take this kind of ownership of your life, things tend to feel better. I've leaned heavily towards personal responsibility in my own life (*most of the time*).

And, most of the time, this perspective does *feel* better. It allows me to be the driver in my own life. Which lends to more agency. I find it's a way more effective and enjoyable way to live life.

It has been a delicate line to walk, at times, with clients.

Because multiple things can be true at once.

Sometimes, the work is to stop minimizing and denying past experiences. It's necessary to acknowledge and validate the reality of a hard experience - maybe even an experience of being a victim to something or someone.

At the same time, knowing that taking personal responsibility for how you choose to move forward can be an incredibly empowering experience. "Victim" does not become your identity.

**This thing happened *to* me. And, it does not *define* me.**

However, not everyone pushing for "personal responsibility" is doing it with benevolent intentions. In an early chapter of this book, I mentioned high-control groups. I spoke about how the concept of taking "personal responsibility" can be weaponized against people. I've also seen this play out in spiritual communities as well as romantic relationships. Taking a grain of truth about the benefits of taking personal responsibility and using it against someone with malicious intent.

**This is where I want you to activate your discernment superpowers - even more.**

It's incredibly powerful to discern when it's appropriate to take ownership for your side of the fence and when something is not yours to own.

Whether it's with a partner, family member, friend, co-worker, boss, therapist, personal development group, spiritual community, or high-control group.

Slowing down and getting really honest with yourself about what is necessary to take personal responsibility for and what parts are not yours to own. You can make yourself "un-gaslightable" by building up these particular discernment muscles.

And these muscles are really important. Because, as humans, we're wired for connection, belonging, and community. And when these muscles are strong, we're much better equipped to thrive in relationships.

It's the foundation for healthy interdependence.

[ 89 ]

# HYPER-INDEPENDENCE

*Do you think it's possible to seek guidance from someone outside of you and still cultivate more trust in yourself?*

**I do.**

I'm not going to speak in circles or leave this one up for reader's interpretation.

> **I want to be crystal clear that *The Self-Trust Model* is not intended to create more islands of hyper-independent people navigating life alone - consulting *only* their inner compass for all life decisions.**

We're pack animals after all. We're social and relational creatures. Connection is our lifeline. Our decisions impact others. And maybe, we don't *have* to learn absolutely every single lesson the hard way!

If it feels like I'm really hammering this point in, it's because I am. It's the biggest lesson my *Fiercely Independent Past Self* refused to learn. And even when she conceded that this is a good lesson for "other people", she still had no intentions of applying the lesson to her own life. Apparently with this lesson, I *did* have to learn it the hard way.

But you don't *have* to be as stubborn as I was.

> (Or maybe, depending on your attachment style, *Life-Scripts,* and past relationships - you're also adamant about proving this lesson wrong. If that's true, I bow to the part of you working tirelessly to keep you safe. *I see you.* )

Regardless, for those of you who are open to learning more, I'm going to continue...

You can have rock solid Self-Trust, but if you don't develop the muscle of trusting yourself to trust others – **your golden skeleton key is essentially useless.**

You can have rock solid Self-Trust, but if you don't develop the muscle of trusting yourself to trust others – **life will always fall flat.**

You'll always be missing out on the magic that's possible when you put your trust in someone who *has* earned it.

I mentioned attachment styles earlier. This isn't a comprehensive guide to learning your attachment style. You'll have to do that somewhere else. But I do want to note that, depending on your attachment style, your growth edge around Self-Trust/trusting others will be different. Just like the attachment styles have a nuanced spectrum, so do these growth edges. But simply put, it looks a bit like this:

. . .

**More Anxiously Attached** = More Ease Putting Trust in Others (even those who *haven't* earned it) & More Difficulty Trusting Yourself

**More Avoidantly Attached** = More Ease Trusting Yourself & More Difficulty Putting Trust in Others (even those who *have* earned it)

Start by just noticing where you may fall on this spectrum and where your edge may be.

## [ 90 ]
# TAROT & SELF-TRUST

*Do you think it's possible to seek guidance from something outside of you and still cultivate more trust in yourself?*

Once again... I'll be very clear, I do.

In fact, when you create and apply a vetting process to taking in input from the outside, you've found yet another way to strengthen your discernment muscles. You're then able to generalize the process to any situation when you're receiving external information.

This chapter is going to focus on one specific way to seek external guidance. But you can apply it to anything outside of yourself. The same principles apply.

*So, grab a cup of tea. And let's talk about tarot.*

Actually, we'll be exploring both tarot and oracle card decks. And how you can use them to build *more* trust with yourself.

---

**Using cards with this intention is *not* about:**

- Fortune telling
- Witchcraft
- Turning over your power
- Religion (or even spirituality)

**The purpose is to leverage an external stimulus to connect you more deeply with the thoughts, beliefs, feelings, and soul whispers already living inside you.**

Over-simplified - it's like flipping a coin to make a decision. Your reaction to the "answer" gives you way more information about yourself, regardless of if it lands on heads or tails.

**Choosing a Deck:**

There are hundreds, if not thousands, of oracle/tarot decks to choose from. If possible, I encourage people to visit a store that has physical decks you can hold and flip through. That way, you can see the designs. You can get a feel for how the shape, size, and texture of the cards feel in your hands. You can shuffle them. You can allow yourself to be drawn towards certain decks. If that's not possible, you can still do your research online and order a deck (or a few).

The main point I want to make here is that you can already begin to have the intention to connect more to yourself - even in the *choosing* of a deck. Notice how your body, soul, and younger parts respond to the images. Trust the pull you have towards a certain card deck, even if it doesn't make logical sense. *Even if none of this makes logical sense.*

. . .

**Connecting with the Deck:**

When you first open your deck, spend some time shuffling. Get a sense for how they feel in your hands. What I've seen is we all end up with our own unique way of shuffling. Just allow some space for this to naturally happen. There's no right way.

**Choosing a Card:**

There are infinite "spreads" you can use when pulling a card(s). Here are just a few ideas to get you started. Use them as a jumping off point for your creativity and curiosity.

- **Daily Message from Self**
  - Every morning ask your capital "S" - Self for a message that you need to hear that day and pull a card for guidance.
- **Tea Talks**
  - Similar to inviting your fears to tea, ask for a message from any of your parts (exiles, managers, firefighters) and pull a card for guidance.
- **Unknown + Known**
  - Pull one card to represent what is currently hidden from your conscious awareness. Pull a second card to represent the aspects of the same situation you're consciously aware of.
- **Soul Whisper + Grounded Action**
  - This is one of my favorite spread ideas from the *Starseed Oracle Deck by Rebecca Campbell.*
  - The first card represents your soul whisper and the second card represents the grounded action step for you to take.
- **Past, Present, Future**
  - Draw 3 cards - one representing each moment in time.

- **Specific Guidance from Self**
    - This one returns to Self energy. When you're struggling with a specific choice point, you can pull one card and ask your Self for guidance on what to consider when making the decision.

**Connecting with Yourself:**

Most decks come with a corresponding book or guide that provides the meaning of each card. Before you ask for someone else's interpretation, I encourage you to first connect to yourself and notice your reaction to the card. Once you've selected your card(s), explore these prompts:

- *How does my body respond to the image and word of the card?*
- *What part(s) of me get activated seeing the word or image?*

Once you've had a chance to notice and sit with your reaction to the card(s), you may want to spend some time writing about what you noticed. You can use the card pull as a journaling prompt and see where your writing exploration takes you.

On some card pulls, you may choose to reveal the meaning of the card according to the guide included. After reading the interpretation, you can follow the same process and notice what arises in you from reading the external information. You can take note of what resonates and what doesn't. It can be another jumping off point for more writing and reflection.

---

As with any new practice you're bringing into your life, it's helpful to set a specific amount of time you want to try it out. Maybe you start with one week or one month of daily card pulls. Then, at the end of that timeframe, check back in with yourself.

- *What did you notice?*
- *How does your connection to yourself feel?*
- *Do you enjoy the practice?*
- *Does it feel helpful?*
- *Do you feel more/less connection to your intuition?*
- *Did you notice yourself wanting an "answer" from the cards?*

For me, I've noticed that this is a seasonal practice. There are times when I am more consistent with pulling cards to connect with my inner wisdom. And times when it gets put on the backburner.

---

Finally, if you notice that this is a practice that deeply resonates with you, here's another idea. Make your own oracle deck.

### Create-Your-Own-Deck

One of my favorite decks I own has prominent women and feminine archetypes throughout history and across many cultures. The corresponding guide shares the story of each woman/deity/goddess along with an inspirational message offered by selecting it.

During one of the groups I offered, I decided to create my own deck to share with the women in the program. Instead of the historical figures, I thought about the many women in my own life who have inspired me, challenged me, and who embody the spirit of Self-Trust. I reached out to them and asked them to share their wisdom around Self-Trust. To share how they have been able to trust themselves more and the impact of trusting their intuition. The *Inspiration Deck* was created.

From there, I also encouraged the women in the program to create their own oracle deck. And you can do the same. Personalized to you. With people you know. With people who've been impactful on your journey. It can also include animals, lessons, gemstones, fictional characters, folklore, cities, seasons, etc. You create your deck - personalized to you. With the images and symbolism that are significant to you.

---

**Hang tight... the *You Can Trust Yourself Oracle Deck* will be here soon...**

# [ 91 ]
# KNOW YOURSELF CHALLENGE

As you read in the last chapter, almost anything can be used as a prompt for reflection.

> **Treat self-reflection like a hammer and start looking at everything as a nail.**

And also... journaling is a straightforward and often illuminating way to know yourself better. So I'd be remiss if I didn't offer some structure for traditional reflection prompts.

Because historically, truths that I wasn't even consciously ready to see yet, have found a way to cryptically reveal themselves to me on pages meant for "my eyes only". And especially on the pages marked for "immediate burning".

When I told you the story of meeting my stubborn intuition on the long anniversary hike with my then-husband, I painted a picture of being blindsided by this discovery of impending divorce.

*Because that's how it felt in the moment.*

It wasn't until much later, as I was reading journals from months before our Pacific Northwest adventure that I saw the clues. And in hindsight - *they were obvious*. I was able to see the writing on the wall as I read about the spiraly abyss I felt myself reluctantly swirling into.

As I continued reading, I remembered the temporary work-around I was convinced could be a long term solution to a marriage of unfortunate incompatibility.

"The Answer", I'd discovered, was to move to Canada for three months - without my husband.

And then, back to our home together for a few months. And then head out again, solo, for a while. You get the idea...

My body experienced the fullest exhale possible as I clicked "buy" on the Airbnb website. I thought I'd finally discovered the way to compromise on the uncompromisable. I smugly thought I'd found a way for us to make "us" work. And I was pretty proud of myself. Even if I still wasn't prepared to look at the fact that compromising on having children wouldn't be as simple as paying for an extended stay in a foreign country.

**If only lying to yourself about your deepest and truest desires for life could actually make them go away...**

Reading my own words many months later offered insight and necessary perspective. I was able to understand why I'd be spiraling so much. I better grasped what had happened to me on that now infamous (only to me) hike. I was able to have understanding and compassion for the part of me that didn't want to see the full truth. The part of me that wanted to get creative about life and put on blinders to anything that could threaten what I thought I wanted.

This is why taking intentional time to slow down and connect to yourself is pivotal in trusting yourself. With consistency and *Radical Honesty*, maybe you'll be able to make proactive decisions from the insights gained. Or maybe the wisdom you discover through these reflection prompts will help you make sense of things in hindsight. Connect the dots looking backwards.

Either way, I know I find both immensely valuable.

That's why I'm offering this challenge to you...

The **Know Yourself Challenge** is 30 days of curated reflection prompts sent directly to your inbox each morning.

I encourage you to take the daily prompt with you on a sunrise stroll each morning. Use it as a jumping off point for self-reflection and allow the bilateral movement of walking to support your brain in finding new connection points. And maybe even a few "aha moments" of clarity.

If nothing else, you'll get some morning sunlight and movement. Two of your five regulation areas for the day - done.

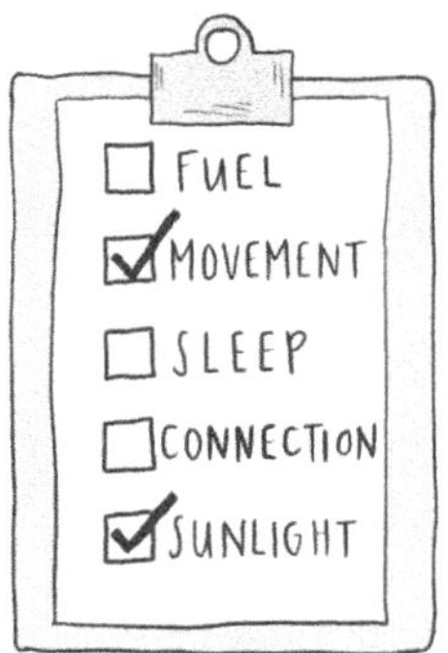


You can also allow your mind to wander with the prompt on your drive to work. Or sit down - putting pen to paper with each morning prompt. However you choose to do it is perfect. Maybe try out a few "styles" of reflecting until you find the one that works best for you.

Just stick with it for the entire challenge, because...

If you're **Radically Honest** with yourself on each prompt...

At the end of 30 days, you'll **Know Yourself** better...

You'll have 30 more reps in **Keeping Promises** to yourself...

And if you choose the sunrise stroll option, you'll have more access to **Regulation** in your nervous system.

You'll be well on your way to **Trusting Yourself More**.

Get instant access to the 30-day Know Yourself Challenge:

## [ 92 ]

# PATHWAYS WE DON'T CHOOSE

You may have been left with the impression from the "Many Paths" chapter that discovering your *Pathways to Self-Trust* is as simple as choosing from a buffet of appealing options such as: embodiment practices, traveling solo, taking a Reiki training, learning to cook, hiking, spiritual exploration, or taking up knitting.

**But, let's be clear, that's a wildly incomplete picture.**

Because we're all going to experience things in life we don't choose.

- Things you'd never want...
- Moments you'd never wish for...
- Experiences you'd bargain with the universe to take back...

They are all going to happen.

I can't promise you a path to genuine confidence lined with only intentional decisions and deliberate pathways you'd *want* to choose. That's not at all been my experience.

**It was the pathways I never wanted, that ultimately led me where I wanted to go.**

---

In "The 13 Lessons" book, I wrote about one way that trust forms between people:

> *"Trust isn't just built in happy and supportive moments. Deeply rooted trust actually forms during the discomfort of real and honest conversations. It's strengthened when we go through challenging times together. Running from hard conversations actually keeps us from the closeness and intimacy we crave."*

The same is true for developing trust with yourself. It's strengthened when you go through challenging moments you never would've volunteered for.

Maybe not always. And maybe not right away.

But it *is* possible to build even more trust with yourself by going through the hardest moments of your life.

This is another reason I can't prescribe you a *Pathway to Self-Trust*. Because I don't know what hardships you're going to face in life. I don't know what devils you'll have to contend with. I don't know what dark nights you'll have to survive.

But even if I could, I wouldn't prescribe (*or wish*) the pathways I didn't choose, on you.

While I want to give you an example to ground this important point home, it also kills me to reduce the worst thing that ever happened to me down to a single bullet point. And trying to capture two decades of shame into another bullet point, feels impossible. The alternative to the bullet points, however, would be full books on both in an attempt to do them justice. We don't have time for that. So bullet points it is...

- For two decades, I dealt with vaginismus and chronic pelvic pain. Long before anyone knew what this was. I felt broken, insecure, alone, and hopeless as I navigated a medical system without answers -and a heavy prescription of gaslighting. A painful journey I tried to wish away my entire life - *eventually* (and painfully) led me into a deeper connection with myself, my body, my voice, my power, and my autonomy. I now have an unshakeable trust in the wisdom of my body and the messages she shares with me. It's a language I probably never would've cared to learn of my own volition.
- The first person I loved after my divorce - died tragically. Grief and despair made me lose absolutely *all* of my fucks. It was that loss of fucks that ultimately led to a kind of confidence I'd never experienced before. My first taste of feeling *truly* confident in myself after decades of deep insecurity - came with a price tag that was way too high. I eagerly bargained with the universe, trying to give it back. Magical thinking at its finest.

Both of these experiences in my life fundamentally shaped me and my ability to trust myself. **I did not want either one**

**of them.** My human form never would've chosen them. They were the hardest things I've ever gone through.

**The pathways we don't choose can have just as much of an impact as the paths we do.**

*Side note: If this is starting to feel a little too "Everything happens for a reason!" - you'll want to check out lesson #8 in my first book.*

What I've seen in my work with hundreds of people, is how an experience in life can become one of the "Crisis of Trust" moments we talked about earlier. But it can also become an *Unwanted Pathway to Self-Trust.*

- Betrayal from a spouse
- Traumatic birth experience
- Chronic illness
- Getting fired
- Questioning parts of your identity
- Starting a business... and failing
- Experiencing a medical mystery
- Death of a loved one
- Getting a cease and desist letter

You didn't choose the terrible, unspeakable, unfathomable thing that happened to you. And for a while, it might disconnect you even further from yourself. It may lead you to doubt yourself and second guess every decision you've ever made. And lead you into a spiral-y abyss of insecurity.

**Stay there as long as grief demands...**

"Winter" as long as you need to...

In my experience, grief doesn't like to be rushed. She will take as long as she takes. And she'll circle back often - even when you thought she was done with you. Don't fight it.

And...

You can also explore how, in the aftermath of the terrible, unspeakable, unfathomable thing that you didn't choose, you can use the rubble to pave a pathway.

A pathway to connecting to yourself - *even deeper than before.*

A pathway to trusting yourself - *more than you ever thought possible.*

[ 93 ]

# THINGS YOU'D NEVER CHOOSE

One way to better understand the unwanted pathways to more Self-Trust you've explored is to create a list of *"Things You'd Never Choose"* or *"How I Lost All My Fucks"*.

It's simple.

Just create a list - of all the things you've experienced in life that you never would've chosen for yourself - that *actually* ended up making you trust yourself more.

I shared my two big ones in the last chapter.

But this list isn't exclusive to a decades-long battle with chronic pain or unexpected death. Also include the minor missteps and frustrations life has thrown at you.

***When has life thrown "life" at you?***

***And who did you become on the other side?***

## [ 94 ]

# WHAT MAKES A GOOD VALUE?

I've already alluded to the importance of identifying and living by your values many times throughout this book. And it's a common suggestion in the personal growth world as well in the mental health space. Some might even suggest doing these exercises early on in your work. But I saved it for the Winter because my hope is, the earlier seasons and chapters have allowed you to build a solid foundation and you're now ready to explore your core values to a greater depth than would've been possible in the Spring.

There are many good reasons why "values work" is so popular.

I would actually venture to say that:

**Living a life aligned with your values is the most direct path to a meaningful life.**

I almost wrote that it's what allows you to live with integrity - but that just shows my bias towards *my* values. Assuming you also value integrity as much as I do.

But that's the thing about values.

Values are not universal. We don't automatically value the same things to the same degree. Values aren't necessarily "good" or "bad". Depending on the *Life-Scripts* we've been operating from, especially from religion and your family of origin, we'll have different values and a different prioritization of values.

**Backing up a little bit, I encourage you sit with these two questions first:**

- *What is a value?*
- *What makes a "good" value?*

**Here's how I define values:**

> Values are what you find meaningful in life. They represent your beliefs about what is most important to you. They are both practical and aspirational.

**Things I think make a "good" value:**

- Clear definition
  - Stating that you value "Family" means different things to different people. Get clear about what the word or phase means to you.
- Limited number
  - There are hundreds of values you could identify. It's impossible to prioritize all of the values - especially when some will naturally conflict with each other.
  - In order to live a life from your values, you have to choose which are the most important.
- Timeless

    - They don't change from morning to night. And they don't change just because you're hungry or tired.
- Direct your choices
    - They can be used as the "guard rails" for *your* actions and behaviors. Not to be mistaken for a measuring stick for others.

## Values Identification + Exploration

Question to consider when identifying your values:

- *What really matters to you?*
- *How do you want to spend your time on this planet?*
- *What kind of person do you want to be?*
- *How do you want to be remembered by the people who knew you best?*
- *On your deathbed, what will you be most proud of?*
- *What makes a meaningful life?*

I encourage you to take time to see what responses naturally arise from within to these questions.

Then, if you want to explore further, you can search through lists of values. These are easy to find anywhere on the internet. Search for "list of values" and you'll find hundreds of values listed out with definitions.

Again, this is when I encourage you to use these lists only as a jumping off point.

Notice how your body responds when you read the words "Achievement", "Compassion", "Freedom", "Wealth", and "Justice". Your response helps you discern what values are most important to you.

*What value do you feel drawn to?*

*What values do you feel indifferent to?*

*What values do you feel an aversion to?*

All of this is information for you to *Know Yourself* better.

Coming back to the limited number, I encourage you to identify your top 5 values. List them out and then consider for each value:

- *How did I come to prioritize this value?*
- *Did I inherit this value from someone or somewhere?*
- *Is this value connected to a Life-Script I've been handed?*
- *How do I express this value in my daily life?*

And a question I think is especially important if you want to be radically honest with yourself...

> **Would someone observing my life know that I value,** (insert your value here)**, based on the way I'm living?**

This is the question that illuminates if you're actually living by your values or if you are using them as a way to signal your virtues.

I can *say* that I value curiosity and intentionality, but if I'm walking around on autopilot passing judgment on everyone I meet - I'm not *actually* living by my stated values.

And it's this incongruence between a stated value and how you're actually living that I've seen cause the most painful and destructive inner turmoil. It causes physical bodies to shut down, mental health issues to arise, and spirals into existential crises to commence.

**Here's what I've discovered for myself about the importance of congruency...**

If my options are either:

- Act in alignment with my values (*even when people may not agree and I may lose them from my life*) or...
- Act in conflict with my values (*but get to keep certain people in my life*)...

I've never regretted making a decision aligned with my values. Because I understand why I made the choice I did. I know the decision is aligned with the kind of person I strive to be. Even when it causes myself and others discomfort. This path does not equate to an "easy path" and it is often filled with grief, but the grief of losing someone from my life is less painful for this particular inner pain of incongruency.

---

I want to offer you an example, but first, let's talk about personal values vs. family values vs. community values.

The way that I've been explaining values so far has primarily been through the lens of identifying your own personal values. Your values as an individual. But as we've talked about throughout this book - we are relational creatures. We're not meant to be islands. So how do we explore our personal values within a broader context of family and/or community values?

Well... as with most things... it depends.

Depending on your *Life-Scripts* from family, religion, political parties, and other communities - your values may have already been prescribed to you. You may have been provided a list of values that do, if fact, work for you.

If that's the case, you may have a strong support system, family, and community around you that share your values. This allows for inner and external congruency.

---

My husband and I did not come together with a shared sense of values passed down from religion, family, or a shared community. So we had to create our own.

**We had to choose and codify our own family values.**

We did this so we could have a shared language, a shared decision-making framework, and a way to hold each other accountable when we fall short of who we aspire to be.

It wasn't a short or easy process. We spent many months sharing our individual values and exploring where our values naturally intersected. When there appeared to be misalignment, we had to bring in the guidance of *The Self-Trust Compass*.

First, by practicing our emotional *Regulation* skills - attempting to not overreact to the "wrong" values in the other person. Then, digging even deeper and practicing *Radical Honesty* with ourselves about what the value *really* is. Though this process, we often discovered there was actually more alignment than initially appeared.

Eventually, we were able to create the list of our top family values. The values that we strive to live from and instill in our children. The values we can lean on when we're struggling with how to make a decision. They're structured in a way that acknowledges the both/and realties of the world.

For example, one of our values is:

**We never give up, but know when to pivot.**

If you remember the *Keep Promises* chapter, you already understand this one. You know the value in following through and doing what you say you're going to do. And also... knowing when to pivot is a discernment superpower. It's more than just stating we value "Persistence".

This structure works for us. You have to decide what works for you. As an individual, as a family unit, or as another type of community you're involved in.

But having shared language and "buy-in" to the value system is powerful.

---

I said I would give you an example of how to use your values as a way to guide your decisions. Here's an example from my own life when I leaned on our family values...

I was navigating a difficult situation with a childhood friend. I was tempted to return to a younger version of myself in the interaction. I felt the part of me who wanted to caretake by being easy, understanding, and overly-validating to the other person, step forward. This part of me wanted to appease the other person and not share my own feelings or thoughts. It felt "easier" and more familiar to just tend to their needs.

But, as I navigated a stone labyrinth in the woods, I thought about how I wanted to respond to this person that was actually aligned with my values. And it was this value that continued to arise in my heart:

> **We always tell the truth, but deliver it with kindness.**

The caretaking part of me wasn't intentionally trying to lie. But as I got deeper into the center of the labyrinth, I realized my habit of minimizing my own experiences to make others feel seen - was a form of being untruthful. Which in turn, makes me untrustworthy - regardless of the intentions of my white lies.

I walked with my value of truth and honesty for a while longer. Knowing what I needed to do.

And, as I began my winding exit from the labyrinth, I rehearsed how to share the truth - with kindness. Because that was just as important to me. I don't value being an asshole. I don't value the sentiment of, **"This is MY truth and if you can't handle it – too bad!!"**

My execution of delivering the truth with kindness is up for debate. I don't fully know how it actually landed for the other person. But I do know I was thoughtful and intentional with why and how I shared my feelings with them.

Without a stated value to lean on at that moment, I might have let my caretaking part override and make my decision. And my guess is, she would have led me down a much longer path of frustration, resentment, and ongoing inner conflict.

[ 95 ]

# I'M NOT GETTING RID OF YOU

The process of consciously exploring and identifying your core values is important because without shining the flashlight around, you'll likely end up with a set of values chosen *for* you. The same way *Life-Scripts* were handed to you.

They will become your operating system without you even knowing it. The same way that "hard work" became mine.

The writing of this book has provided me an opportunity to get to know my hard working part. We've spent many mornings having tea together. *She loves a splash of eggnog in hers.* These tea times have helped me come to understand just how deeply engrained the value of hard work has been in my family - for many generations back.

As trust grew, she shared more. Eventually pulling back the curtain completely - showing me how she'd been subconsciously running my entire life. Making all my decisions. She even got good at masquerading as "Self". She was proud of herself. And relieved to finally share it with someone.

*Damn, she's good.*

I had to admit, I was impressed. The web of choices she was involved in spinning was even bigger, and more intricate, than I'd imagined.

So when I began to question her - her defensiveness made sense. When I began to wonder out loud if it was *absolutely true* that she was the *only* reason for any success in life. She immediately had receipts to show me. Reminding me of everything I'd ever gotten in life because of the hard work put into getting it.

My hard working part had been working hard my whole life - and she understandably wanted credit for it.

**Thank you, Thank you, Thank you.**

Just as I have immense gratitude for my ancestors' hard work. I have immense gratitude for my own hard working part. For all she's done for me. Even when she tricked me into thinking I was operating from Self energy. I understand her motives. And I'm eternally grateful for her.

**Thank you, Thank you, Thank you. And I promise, I'm not trying to get rid of you.**

One risk in identifying *Life-Scripts* or coming to realize an indoctrinated value has been running your life, is the impulse to immediately reject it. To label it as "bad" because you didn't choose it. You may want to do the "opposite" of whatever value or script was thrust upon you.

But if you remember from the *Life-Scripts* chapters:

- Unconsciously following the *Life-Scripts* you were handed isn't choice.
- However, unconsciously rebelling and doing the opposite of the *Life-Scripts* you were handed, also, isn't choice.

It all comes back to choosing with intention.

Once I realized how expertly my hard working part had been running the show (*aka: my life*), I'll admit, I did have an initial reaction to make it stop. **I wanted to separate my value and my worth from my ability to work hard.**

But sitting with it a bit longer, my reaction revealed itself to be another part - *not* Self.

This part *also* made sense to me.

The process of unblending from all my parts continued. Unblending from the hard working part. Unblending from the part that wanted to get rid of the hard working part.

On and on... until gradually - and then all at once - more clarity emerged.

This **clarity** - indicating that I was getting more and more access to Self energy.

And Self had some simple yet profound wisdom to share with these previously tunnel-visioned parts of mine:

- It doesn't have to be either/or. Working hard has absolutely allowed me to reach certain dreams and goals I've had in life. I get to be grateful for the value of hard work being engrained in me. I even get to consciously *choose* hard work as a value now. And - hard work is not the *only* ingredient for success.

- There is something profound waiting for me when I learn how to find "ease" in my business and life. There is something powerful waiting for me when I choose the path of things I'm good at - instead of constantly choosing the "hardest" path.

All of this clarity from Self continued to bubble up in my conscious mind. And I realized, **hard work was never the enemy**. Because let's be real, if hard work was actually the enemy to overcome - you wouldn't be reading this book right now.

Hard work had actually been conflated with something else. And it was the glorification of this "something else" that was the real issue.

The question was never, *"Have I worked hard enough to deserve this success?"*

The unconscious question engrained in the dark corners of my psyche...

The vetting process indoctrinated into the cells of my body...

The karmic wound that had been running the show was...

**"Have I suffered enough to be deserving?"**

[ 96 ]

# DREAM INTEGRATION

There's another world, but it's in this one.
- Paul Eluard

"*Dreamland*" - as we call it in our family - can be a liminal portal to another abyss. It can feel sweet and intoxicating - tempting you to stay a while longer... willing you back to slumber.

Other nights, it can trap you in spaces where demons hide.

Regardless of if the alternate reality is one you want to soak in or escape as quickly as possible - *Dreamland* can feel like you're straddling two worlds.

Disorienting you on your return journey home.

In that way, it's just like any other non-ordinary state of consciousness (NOSC).

**NOSC is just like what it sounds - a state of consciousness that* *is not ordinary. A state that is altered - different from an ordinary waking consciousness.*

That's what I'm talking about in this book when I write about the principles of psychedelic therapy. The *Self-Trust Model* looks at how preparation and integration for mystical journeys can be applied to *any* non-ordinary state of consciousness.

No substances required.

**Consider, what are some ways you can access a NOSC without drugs?**

*I'm not prescribing any of these ideas to you, but this list might help get your creative juices flowing...*

- Breathwork
- Meditation
- Silence retreat
- Sensory deprivation
- Fasting
- Binaural beats
- Hiking deep into the woods and sitting in nature for an extended period of time
- Hypnosis
- Tantric sex practices
- Dancing/Music
- Dreaming

I once heard it said that dreams are like letters from your unconscious mind. And if you don't take time to notice and reflect on your dreams, it's like leaving the letter unopened in your mailbox.

Intentionally creating a practice of opening the letters from your unconscious mind every morning can be a path to trusting yourself more. It's a way to learn more about yourself and what's being processed in the background of your psyche. A way to connect to the different parts of yourself.

I've been interested in dreams to varying degrees throughout my life. Sometimes, doing my own research, looking at the meaning and significance of symbols in dreams. I treated it the same way I encouraged you to treat the tarot + oracle practices. Not to turn over your power to a dream interpretation book, but to use it as a catalyst to your own inner wisdom.

The dream interpretation books can be an interesting gateway into the space of connecting to your dreams, and ultimately, connecting to hidden parts of yourself.

That being said, I've also had periods in my life when I required something more.

During a "dark night of the soul" time in my life, my dream life was intense - to say the least. I was feeling lost, and honestly a little scared, with what was happening in my psyche on the nights I was able to find sleep.

I needed more support than an internet search on *"dreams with men dressed in black holding guns coming for me"* could provide.

So I reached out to my dream guy.

My *actual* dream guy - a friend of mine who's a Jungian analyst. He has deep wisdom about the archetypes of dreams, common themes in trauma survivors, and was able to shine a light on things in my dreams I hadn't yet paid attention to. He sent me resources to read, ideas to consider, and tools to help me remember my dreams.

It was a process.

But over the course of a year or so, "light" came back to my dreams. Literal light. I still remember the feeling after the first time there was sunlight in my dreams again. For nearly a year, my dreams had been scary and filled with death. Even the dreams that were hopeful and playing out alternate realities I wished were true - they were all still literally dark. It was always night time.

**Grief is synonymous with the cold and dark winters of our life.**

It's falling between worlds for a while - while the veil is thin.

As the book, *Wintering* by *Katherine May,* encourages us to do - I learned to invite the winter in. And allow for the possibility of wisdom *inside* the winter.

Eventually, just like every snowy season I've ever experienced, the ice melts. The days eventually get longer. And one morning, I woke up to the realization that it had been daylight outside the window in my dreams. The first sign of Spring.

---

Dreams are a delicate dance of discernment. Knowing when to connect inward for the message. Knowing when you can open the letter from your unconscious mind alone. And knowing when to seek guidance outside of you - from an interpretation book, a friend, a therapist, a partner, a coach, or your own personal "dream guy".

[ 97 ]

# DOORS

I took myself on a writing retreat to Portland, Oregon to finish the first draft of this book. The forest of the PNW is where my love of hiking first intersected with writing. During the same dark night of the soul that led to never-ending death dreams - writing became my way through. The two are forever intertwined now - making up the strands of my DNA.

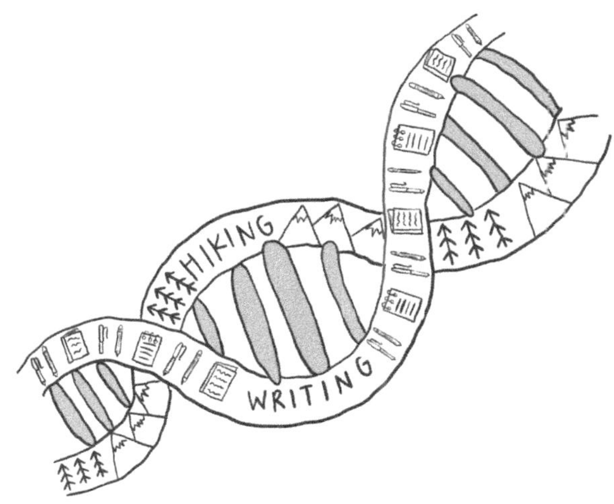

Grief ripped me open in unimaginable ways, the way only grief can. And the only path forward involved long treks into the forest alone and writing an entire book in the 2nd person. *A book that will forever be "For My Eyes Only"...*

I reached a point in the writing of the book you're currently reading that I needed some distraction-less time to make the progress I knew was right on the edge of my fingertips. And I immediately knew where I needed to escape to.

During this trip to the "City in the Forest" I was staying at one of those Airbnb's that has a private room, but shared living space. These arrangements are not my preferred way to travel, but my budget as a writer is different than it was when I lived in Portland as a traveling therapist who had an excuse to pay a premium for privacy.

That housing backstory is relevant only to paint a picture for you of how many doors there were where I was staying. A front door, a door to the main house, a door to the bathroom, a door to the room I was staying in, a door to the other private rooms. Lots and lots of doors.

I woke the first morning with memories still lingering from my trip to *Dreamland.* Because the dream happened in the actual space I was opening my eyes to, the liminal in-between space remained longer than normal. I wasn't sure what was "real".

In the dream, there were even more doors than what I was seeing in front of me with wakeful eyes. Doors I hadn't seen before. In the dream, all the doors were open. The door to my private room - now exposed. Front door - wide open. The doors I didn't even know were there - now were off their hinges. Everywhere I look - the doors are open.

The dream had an emotional resonance I didn't understand yet, but couldn't shake.

---

I eventually found myself down a few internet rabbit holes, asking an oracle deck for more clarity about the dream, as well as listening to a long voice note from a (different) "dream friend" with her interpretations of what it all meant.

According to a hodgepodge of different search results, doors are considered one of the oldest recorded dream symbols. A few more interpretations of their symbolism are:

- Doors signify beginnings and transitions in life.
- An open door is an invitation from the unconscious to check out what's beyond it.
- The more doors there are, the more complex the choice might be.
- Doors are metaphorical symbols that encourage you to open or unlock different aspects of your life.
- A door is a portal - acting as an entrance or exit. Metaphorically, a door can lead to almost anything - another world, a new beginning, a challenge or an opportunity.
- When closed - keeping us from being able to cross, locking us in. Maybe protecting us; *but maybe trapping us.*
- When open - exposing us to others. Maybe making us vulnerable to attack; *but maybe opening us up to connection.*

This is what stuck out to me in the dream. My initial emotional response in the dream - seeing all the open doors and doors off their hinges - was fear. It felt dangerous to be so exposed. But as the dream progressed, I realized that I wasn't *actually* in danger. All the exposure, all the visibility, *wasn't* a true threat to me.

---

As much as I appreciated my friends' take in her voice notes and the interpretations from the books, ultimately I was led back to my initial reaction to the dream. Other people's words just helped me make sense of what I already felt.

Choosing to end my career as a therapist and pursue writing, was pushing me to be seen by others in a whole new way. I could no longer hide behind the secrecy of my chosen profession. And it was activating the part of me who was terrified of vulnerability leading to being misunderstood. The idea of being more exposed and visible in the dream initially felt dangerous. Just as putting up the first video of me on social media felt existential.

It didn't take long for me to realize, there wasn't actually anything coming to attack me. My body was responding to the perception of threat because it was unfamiliar - *not because it was actually dangerous.*

[ 98 ]

# GIVING + RECEIVING

As we near the end of this book, I want to offer one more practice for you to explore. A practice "given" to me by these magical redwoods inside *Hoyt Arboretum*. Just one of the many gifts offered from the forests of Portland, Oregon.

If you have access to a tree - I encourage you to go outside and have this experience with a real tree. If not, you can visualize this experience in your mind's eye. Bringing to mind the most magnificent tree you can imagine. With a broad and strong trunk.

- Place both hands on the tree.
- Close down your eyes.
- Imagine you are sending love and energy through your right hand into the tree.
- With your left hand, feel and receive the love and energy from the tree.

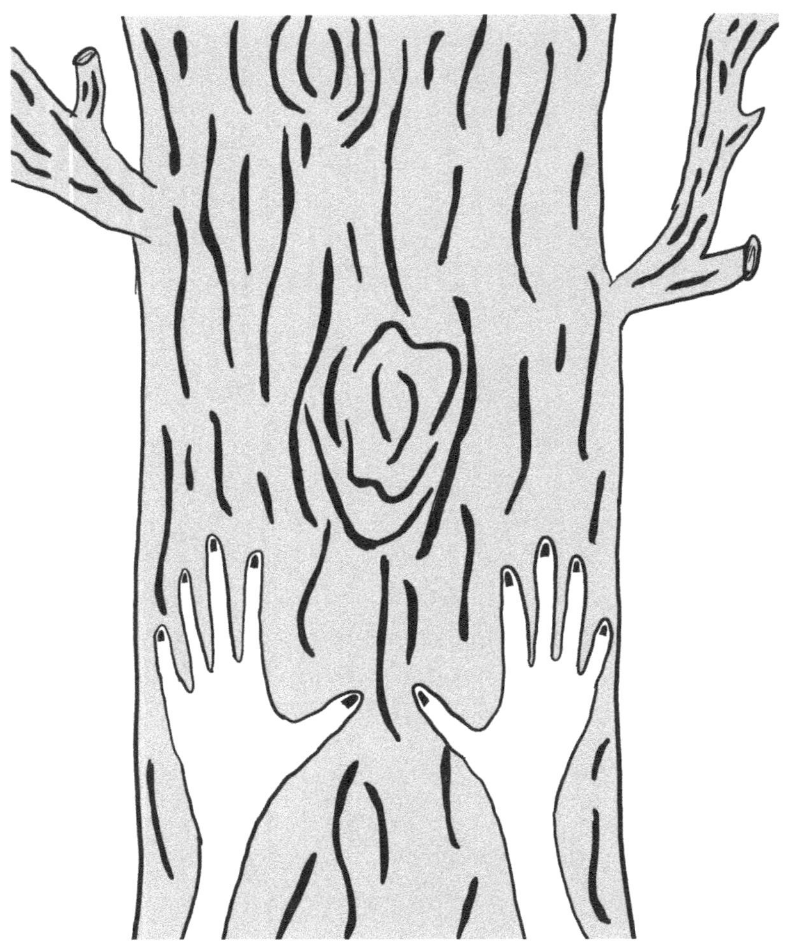

Allow your body, your heart, and spirit to complete the circuit of giving and receiving energy. *From Mother Earth. From The Universe. From You. From Nothing. From Everything.*

[ 99 ]

# "MORE"

I hope this far into the book, you've given yourself permission to desire the life you *actually* want. To look down at the golden skeleton key you're now holding in your hands and be radically honest about the doors you want to open. Whatever those doors happen to look like. Life doesn't have to just be about symptom reduction and survival mode.

**It's okay to want more than "fine."**

Ready for the exciting (*and maybe slightly terrifying*) part?

*You* are the only one who can define what "more" means to you. My "more" might not make any sense to you. My idea of "more" might sound, to you, like a terrible way to do life. In fact my current definition of "more" doesn't even make any sense to me from five years ago.

I can't prescribe my "more" to you.

And you can't just take someone else's recipe for a "good life". You might be allergic to their ingredients.

| SOMETIMES "MORE" MEANS MORE... | AND SOMETIMES "MORE" MEANS LESS... |
|---|---|
| * MORE CONFIDENCE + LOVE | * MORE STILLNESS |
| * MORE FREEDOM | * MORE PEACE |
| * MORE ADVENTURES + FUN | * MORE QUIET |
| * MORE LAUGHTER + PLAY | * MORE SOLITUDE |
| * MORE MOVEMENT | * MORE BREAKS |
| * MORE ABUNDANCE | * MORE REST |
| * MORE SEX + PASSION | * MORE SNUGGLES |
| * MORE THAN JUST GETTING BY | * MORE BLANK SPACE |
| * MORE THAN JUST PAYING THE BILLS ON TIME | * MORE SLOWNESS |
| * MORE THAN JUST OKAY | * MORE NESTING |
| * MORE THAN A "SIMPLE LIFE" | * MORE AFTERNOON NAPS |
| | * MORE OF A "SIMPLE LIFE" |

Defining your "more" requires you to trust yourself. That's why we waited until the end of the book for this definition. You had to work your way around the Self-Trust compass first...

You had to get **Radically Honest** with yourself.

You had to consistently **Keep Promises** to yourself.

You had to find ways to **Regulate** your nervous system.

You had to really get to **Know Yourself**.

Can you feel your discernment muscles getting stronger each time you re-visit a direction on the compass?

Remember, none of this happens immediately. It can be a lifelong process of returning home to yourself and constantly redefining your "more". Over and over again. As many times as necessary in this human existence.

Aaaaaaaand. *Because there's always an "And."*

Throughout this lifelong journey, you don't have to be in a constant state of excavation. Yes, there will likely be many seasons of digging deep into your psyche and doing the healing work to see the changes you want in life.

And sometimes, the only thing the season of life you're in calls for is... living in it. Showing up and being present in the life you've created.

And maybe... having a little fun along the way.

[ 100 ]

# HOLD ONTO YOUR KEY

When I look down now at the golden skeleton key in my hands, I'm reminded of the "doors dream" from a few months ago. Sitting and remembering all the many doors.

> **What if the abundance of doors my subconscious showed me was a representation of all the doors this key has already opened for me?**

I'm filled with gratitude as I reflect on each door this key has turned the lock on:

- The door to *finally* finding true confidence.
- The door to leaving a marriage to chase a life my soul was pulling me towards.
- The door to starting my own business.
- The door to setting necessary boundaries in relationships.
- The door to a kind of love I never could've imagined for myself.

- The door to creating (and then leaving) a dream job.
- The door to becoming a published author - *twice, if you're reading this.*
- The door to chasing the evolving definitions of "more".
- The door to freedom.
- The door to valuing myself for more than just what I can offer to others.
- The door to standing up for myself.
- The door to living a life I deliberately chose.

I'm proud to look down and see the key I'm holding...

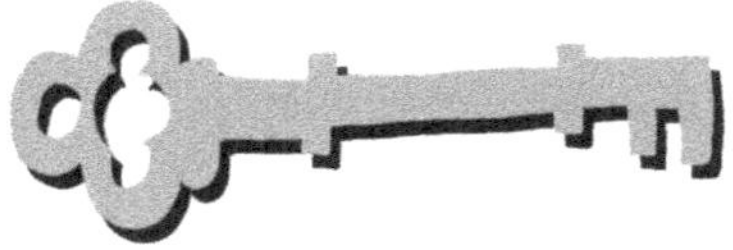

A key that I've worked my ass off to get. Both the grinding and long-hours kind of hard work I was raised to value. And also, the kind of hard work that is dismantling toxic views of hard work and conflating it with suffering.

A kind of hard work that requires rest and true surrender.

**Because what I've learned to be true for me is this:**

> True surrender is required for trust.
>
> Trust and surrender are intrinsically linked.

# THE SUMMIT

January 23rd

I guess if you're reading this... I published another book. Or you somehow got your hands on my personal journals...

Once I realized that's what I was doing... writing a book about The Self-Trust Model - I had ideas about how I thought it "should" end. I thought I knew what would make a "good ending".

In hindsight though, I realize those "endings" werent coming from Self.

They were primarily focused on replacing and then surpassing the revenue from the previous era of my business. Rationalizing that a certain amount of income would make The Self-Trust Model "legit". Which in turn, would make my business legit.

Which in turn, would make me... legit.

Thankfully, through the publishing of my first book and the writing of this book - certain ego-driven parts of me have been able to settle a bit. At least long enough to let Self write the ending.

You see, Self is a wise and steady presence.

She has a bird's eye view. She understands all the "unlocking" that has happened. She grasps the world way beyond numbers in a bank account. She understands purpose, worth, creativity, and the cyclical nature of life.

She doesn't just understand surrender as a concept. She knows how and when to fully embody it. She knows the only ending that makes sense - is at the precipice of the unknown...

At the cusp of "maybe"...

Because, maybe I'll eventually be able to replace my therapy income with my writing.

Maybe, I'll eventually publish the raw and

messy memoir about my indecision around motherhood.

Maybe, I'll return to offering 1-1 work because that's what feels good.

Maybe, I'll run Adventure Club again - the right way.

Maybe, I'll explore another creative project.

Maybe, I'll get to experience pregnancy and the birth portal - now that I know I want it.

Maybe, becoming a mother will be my catalyst into an even deeper connection with my intuition - in ways unfathomable to me now.

Maybe, it took me too long to realize I want to become a mother.

Maybe, I'll have a different initiation.

Maybe, I have other lessons to learn.

Maybe, I'm meant to more fully embody my role as a "bonus mom" and be the best possible Maddy there ever was.

Maybe, I'll reconnect with estranged family members.

Maybe, we can love each other better from a distance in this season.

Maybe, death will once again rock me to my core.

Maybe, there are people I've yet to meet that will forever change my life.

Maybe, I'll visit a place and never want to leave.

Or hell, maybe I'll just go back to waiting tables.

Maybe...

Maybe...

Maybe...

Honestly, maybe I have no fucking idea what lies ahead.

But, no matter what versions of "maybe" manifest, I know I'll be okay...

**That's the "magic" of Self-Trust.**

# KEEP IT GOING

The "Maybe Path" has gotten much clearer in the months since writing the final chapter...

Are you a therapist, life coach, retreat leader, birth worker, yoga teacher, body worker or other service provider?

Want to use *The Self-Trust Model*™ in your practice?

# ACKNOWLEDGMENTS

***Writing a book is not a solo journey...***

To *Taylor*, thank you for always being my biggest hypeman - in writing and life. Thank you for "unlocking" new doors in me. Without a doubt, I would not be here without you. Thank you for patiently showing me, again and again, that it can actually be safe to trust others. Without the lessons we've learned together, crucial elements of trust would still be missing from this book. Thank you for your reverence for the feminine and the magic - *even when you don't understand it.* You make life a wild and beautiful ride.

To *Kashie* and *Journey*, thank you for being my rocks over the past five years. Personally, I don't know where I'd be without you. Surprise custom playlists and curated welcome packages are my love languages. And professionally, I don't think this book would've existed without your never-ending support. From the very literal and practical support in helping me set up (and tear down) the spaces for *Adventure Club. Even when I micromanage it all a bit too much and don't let you help - you were actually always helping.* To the very mystical and unseeable energetic support you've given me through hundreds of hours of conversations, feedback about the model, and encouragement about the writing. Not to mention countless very generous interpretations of card pulls.

To all the women who trusted in me and joined this community, especially all the *Adventure Sisters,* thank you. I don't take your trust lightly.

To *Kasey*, thank you for saying *"Yes!"* to sharing your illustrations with the world. Your "doodles" have always resonated so deeply with me - often more than words alone. This book wouldn't be complete without your art and I'm grateful you chose to take the leap... before you were ready. We are *all* so lucky.

There have been countless women who've supported my writing path that I want to offer gratitude for. Those who cheered me on before my first book launch, provided honest feedback about how to make this book better, wrote a review, shared this book with a friend, hosted a book club with my first book, or joined the BTS squad. If you attended a book signing, a speaking event, or bought my first book – THANK YOU! Your support means more to me than you know. And a special MASSIVE THANK YOU to: *Yaya, Haley, Meghan, Raelynn, Caitlan, Lo, Lily, Sydney, Madison,* and *Ashley*.

And finally, to C & *J*. Thank you for all the love and lessons. This is for you. More than anything, my biggest wish is for you to grow up knowing that ***you can trust yourself.***

---

To reiterate chapter 67... I don't care if the science behind gratitude practices are "real". I only care about how I feel after taking the time to genuinely reflect on each person I just mentioned and the many more who came to mind when sitting down to write this. *Thank you, Thank you, Thank you.*

## ABOUT THE AUTHOR

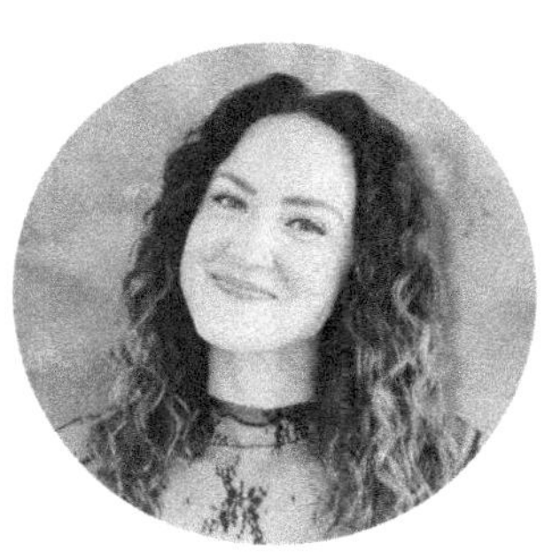

Emily began her career as a therapist in 2010 and founded her private practice, *Curiosity Rising,* in 2019. With a passion for holistic and integrative approaches, she specialized in working with complex trauma and anxiety through the lens of somatics, parts work, and psychedelic therapy.

She's the creator of *The Self-Trust Model*™ A framework designed to empower women to overcome self-doubt, overthinking, and insecurity so they can feel confident chasing their big dreams. She now leads training and certification programs for those interested in applying the model to their practices. You can also learn more about the model on her podcast: *The Self-Trust Podcast.*

Enjoy Emily's first book: *Can People Really Change? 13 Lessons from 13 Years as a Therapist.*

Formerly a proud nomad, Emily now finds solace in home and family amidst the beauty of Colorado. Whether she's hiking in the mountains or forest, it's always after a few tea lattes.

Learn more about current offerings from Emily at:

**www.curiosityrising.com**

# ABOUT THE ILLUSTRATOR

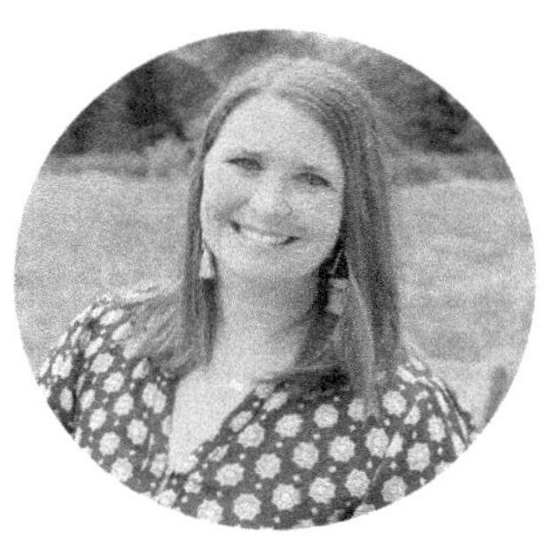

Kasey Strobel is a self-taught artist and illustrator based out of Kansas City, Missouri. As a child, art class was like walking into a magical world of color, art supplies and wonder.

Sadly, adulthood brought a disconnection from her vibrant, creative self. Through meditation, therapy, and motherhood Kasey has ultimately rekindled her love of art.

Today, she views creating as a practice in presence, healing, and slowing down. When not illustrating, she enjoys adventures in nature with her husband and two sons.

To learn more about Kasey and her art visit:

**www.kaseystrobel.com**

## GLOSSARY + INDEX

### SELF-TRUST MODEL

*Adventure Club* – A transformative group coaching experience designed to help women explore Self-Trust, personal growth, and deep connection. Unlike traditional therapy, it includes travel, outdoor activities, and guided conversations to facilitate breakthroughs in confidence and decision-making. This group was the catalyst for codifying *The Self-Trust Model*.

*Golden Skeleton Key* – A metaphor representing Self-Trust as the ultimate tool for unlocking confidence, boundaries, decision-making, meaningful relationships, and overall well-being. Instead of needing separate solutions for different problems, strengthening Self-Trust enables transformation across multiple aspects of life.

*Land of Conjecture* –A conceptual space where assumptions, doubts, and uncertainty cloud decision-making. It represents the mental loops and overthinking patterns that can erode Self-Trust.

*Life-Scripts* – The scripts we've been handed for our performance in life. Often without our conscious awareness, they instruct us on how we should live, love, work, and do life.

*Self-Trust* – A state of deep knowing that you can rely on your own internal compass to handle whatever is thrown at you in life.

*Self-Trust Compass* – A core concept in *The Self-Trust Model,* it represents the four fundamental directions of Self-Trust:

North (Radical Honesty), East (Keeping Promises), South (Regulation), and West (Knowing Yourself). It serves as a practical guide to help individuals navigate their personal and relational journeys.

- *North (Radical Honesty)* – Emphasizes speaking and living one's truth, even when uncomfortable. It requires deep self-awareness and the courage to acknowledge reality without self-deception.
- *East (Keeping Promises)* – Focuses on integrity and follow-through. It emphasizes making and keeping commitments to oneself and others while learning discernment about which promises are worth maintaining and which should be consciously broken.
- *South (Regulation)* – Focuses on nervous system regulation. It emphasizes grounding techniques, nervous system awareness, and self-regulation to build resilience and maintain inner peace.
- *West (Knowing Yourself)* – Encourages self-reflection and authenticity. It involves understanding personal values, beliefs, desires, and past experiences to create a life aligned with one's core Self.

*The Self-Trust Model™* – A structured framework developed by Emily Romero to help individuals overcome self-doubt, overthinking, and insecurity. It integrates elements of psychology, nervous system regulation, and self-reflection to support confident decision-making and personal growth.

*Speed of Trust* – The natural pace at which trust develops in relationships, both with oneself and others. It acknowledges that trust cannot be forced or rushed but is built gradually through consistent actions, honesty, and alignment between words and behaviors.A principle used in *Adventure Club* and personal growth work.

*Titration* – A concept borrowed from somatic therapy, referring to the gradual exposure to emotional or psychological experiences to build resilience and integration without overwhelming the nervous system. In Self-Trust work, titration allows for slow, manageable growth without triggering fear or shutdown.

*Values* - What you find meaningful in life. They represent your beliefs about what is most important to you. They are both practical and aspirational.

## MODERN TOOLS

## THERAPY WISDOM

www.ingramcontent.com/pod-product-compliance
Lightning Source LLC
Chambersburg PA
CBHW051105150425
25159CB00008B/53

* 9 7 9 8 9 9 1 5 6 9 6 3 7 *